6,75

GLOWING B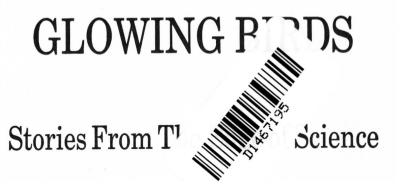DS

Stories From T... Science

Patrick Huyghe

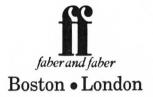

faber and faber

Boston • London

Portions of this book originally appeared in somewhat different form in *Science Digest, Omni, New York, American Way, Psychology Today,* and *The New York Times Magazine.* The author is grateful to these publications for their permission to reprint.

Library of Congress Cataloging in Publication Data

Huyghe, Patrick.
  Glowing Birds.

  1. Biology—Miscellanea. 2. Medicine—Miscellanea.
3. Science—Miscellanea. I. Title.
QH313.H89   1985   081   84–28669
ISBN 0–571–12533–6 (pbk.)

For my parents

To Hugh —
Best future wishes
PW Aw
May 14, 1994

CONTENTS

Introduction

Mind

Life

Universe

Frontiers

INTRODUCTION

A friend once pointed out to me that I seemed fascinated with communicating the strangeness of things. That is true in a sense, but perhaps it's just that I have a different way of looking at the world. We live in an age that focuses its attention on the common, the everyday, the highly visible. We are preoccupied with political power, sex in any form, death when it occurs in large numbers or among the famous, and money in large amounts. I think such a limited view ignores a good deal.

As a consequence, most of the science stories in this book are not the sort you will normally read about. There is nothing here about the space shuttle, about AIDS, or about pollution of the environment. The press covers these topics thoroughly. My concern here is with science stories of another sort, with those on the edge of science.

An edge is an area where things begin or end, so the stories you will find on the edge of science are also of two types. There are those on the forging edge, where the doors of new frontiers are flung wide open, and there are those on the neglected edge, where controversial subjects are scorned or feared by orthodox scientists. Given enough time, one often turns into the other.

The topics you will read about range from the depths of the mind to the furthest reaches of the universe. There are stories about the beginnings of life, of civilization, of writing, of memory, and of artificial minds. There are stories about worlds buried deep within the human mind, worlds ruled by imaginary companions, by nighttime terrors, by odd compulsions and awesome powers. There are stories of life, of invisible amoeba that feast on brain cells, of large ape-like creatures in the

Pacific Northwest, of humans who use their teeth like animals. There are stories about medicine, its miracles and its curses, about plants that heal and machines designed to do the same. And there are stories of the universe, from the monster at the heart of our galaxy to what are perhaps the most poetic and magnificent objects in the cosmos.

—Patrick Huyghe
January 1985

Time is not a road, not a river; it is a room where one notices different things.—W. H. AUDEN

God not only plays dice. He also sometimes throws the dice where they cannot be seen.—STEPHEN W. HAWKING

No matter how unlikely a thing is, if it happens, it happens.—STANISLAW LEM

MIND

FIRST MEMORIES

"My earliest memory is of waking up one morning with blood on my pillow and being very frightened. It seems that I fell off my high chair the night before and hit my head, and during the night there was some bleeding from my skull."

"I don't remember how old I was but I distinctly remember the joy of digging both hands into the dirt and stuffing it into my mouth."

"My first memory is of a chocolate birthday cake with white frosting and pink trim, and a little wooden train chugging around it."

Think back, for a moment, to your own first memory. It is probably not of your mother's face, as you might expect, or of the hands of the doctor in the delivery room. No, more likely the tantalizing event comes from several years later. Perhaps you recall the birth of a sibling. Goethe did. "One of my first memories," the great German poet told Freud, "is of my father sitting on his bed in his nightclothes, laughingly telling me that I had acquired a brother."

That first childhood memory is notoriously hard to pin down. First you must avoid the influence of family photographs and stories you were told about but don't remember personally. While this distinction is easy to understand, in practice it is hard to make. Then, once a truly personal experience has come to mind, you may find it difficult to remember exactly when it happened.

You may even wonder if it happened at all. Jean Piaget used to tell of an early memory in which he had nearly been kidnapped as his nurse was wheeling him down the Champs Elysees in Paris at the age of two. His recollection included the fact that the nurse's face was scratched by the kidnappers during the fracas. But more than a dozen years later, the nurse confessed that she had fabricated the kidnapping story.

Our earliest childhood memories have a magical quality about them, if for no other reason than by virtue of being the apparent beginnings of our conscious lives. These "islands in the sea of oblivion," as the novelist Esther Salaman called them, have fascinated psychologists for more than a century. Their studies of the phenomenon, from Sir Francis Galton's in 1879 to those of the present, indicate that our early memories are remarkably similar in their surface details.

"Almost all of our earliest memories are located in the fourth year of life," says psychologist John Kihlstrom of the University of Wisconsin, "between the third and fourth birthdays." Like previous studies, his survey of 150 high school and college students, conducted with the help of Columbia University psychologist Judith Harackiewicz, showed that most of our early recollections are visual memories and many of them are in color. Their content, however, varies widely, and seems to fall into three broad categories: trauma, transition, and trivia. Other studies have shown that the first memories of women appear to date from a somewhat earlier point in their lives than those of men, but the difference, which may be the result of IQ rather than sex, is tiny, no more than a couple of months.

The pioneers of psychoanalysis attached a great significance to first memories. Freud believed that they contained the key to the secret chambers of a person's life. Alfred Adler accorded them a central place in his school of Individual Psychology. "The first memory will show the individual's fundamental view of life," he said. Adler firmly believed that such memories have great diagnostic value, regardless of whether they are real or imaginary, because of their unique capacity for revealing a person's attitude toward self, others, and life in general.

Autobiographies provide numerous examples of our tendency to fasten onto early experiences that are important to us. Golda Meir's earliest recollection, which she thought may have been a dream, is of a group of Jews being trampled by cossack horses in Czarist Russia. The earliest recollections of Seymour Papert, the creator of the LOGO computer language for children, all have to do with wheels and mechanical things, figuring out what things do and how they work. Albert Einstein remembered receiving a magnetic compass at about the age of four and being awed by the needle's urge to point north.

"Some people think that these early experiences may somehow be formative of personality and that's why they get remembered," Kihlstrom says, "but I don't think that's right." Do our memories make us, or do we make our memories? Has the person become an alcoholic because his first drink was a positive experience, or has the person who is now an alcoholic reconstructed his past to think of that first drink as something positive? "I think that personality leads to a selectivity of memory," says Kihlstrom, "that people remember things that are consistent with the conception they have of themselves."

Early childhood recollections belong to what psychologists call autobiographical memory. Its most salient feature, considering the novelty and richness of childhood experience, is that adults have so few memories from the first several years of life. This poverty in the number of early recollections has been a puzzle to psychologists ever since Sigmund Freud observed the phenomenon in his patients at the turn of the century.

This apparent amnesia, which Freud labelled infantile or childhood amnesia, applies only to our memories about the self, not to our memory for words learned or objects and people recognized. Freud believed that we lose contact with most of our autobiographical memories before the age of six because as children we repress the anxiety-evoking sexual and agressive memories from the Oedipal phase. All that remains, he noted, are "screen memories," memories that are totally lacking in feeling.

"Childhood amnesia does exist, but it's not necessarily Oedipal," contends Emory University professor Ulrich Neisser, who is widely regarded as the father of cognitive psychology. "The child forgets everything about the self, not just sexual or aggressive memories. We begin to remember our life pretty well only from about the age of five or six because that's when we go to school and develop an organized structure for our lives."

But if schooling does help children organize their lives with respect to space and time and allows them to better encode episodes and later retrieve those events from the past, it would seem that those children who attended nursery school would have more childhood memories than those who entered school at the age of five or so. Neisser's own studies, however, have failed to confirm this intriguing hypothesis.

"There is actually no compelling evidence that the phenomenon of childhood amnesia even exists," says Kihlstrom. Some people will report having memories which date before the age of three, and most surveys of childhood memories indicate that there is no sudden drop-off in the number of memories at a certain age. The frequency of memories simply appears to decrease as a function of age.

So perhaps what we call childhood amnesia is really no different than normal forgetting. "After all," says David Rubin, a researcher in human memory at Duke University, "childhood was a long time ago, and perhaps the reason we don't remember much of it is because we have just normally forgotten it. But then again, many of the memories reported to have occurred before the age of three or four are unverified, and perhaps people are filling in memories for this period in their lives because they want a complete life."

People generally assume that the reason they cannot remember anything before about the about the age of three is that they had no memory before that age. Nothing could be further from the truth. "If you look at a three or four year old in action," Neisser says, "you will see a person who remembers quite a lot, in the sense that you can ask a four year old about things that happened the year before and get very intelligent answers. It's not that they have no memory, but when they become ten or twelve or twenty they don't remember those things much anymore."

Since the mid-1970s Marion Perlmutter and her associates at the University of Minnesota's Institute of Child Development have tried to assess the mnemonic abilities of preschool children in both experimental and naturalistic settings. In a study with Chris Todd, she examined the conversations between young children and adults to determine, among other things, the length of time children could retain information. She found that the youngest children, those between two years-eleven months and three years-two months, could retain a memory for events which had occurred more than seven-and-a-half months previously. The older children, those between three years-nine months and four years-six months, could retain information for episodes which had occurred as far back as fourteen-and-a-half months.

"The ability of these children to retain information from such an early age was impressive," notes Perlmutter, "particularly since in some cases they demonstrated a verbal recall for events that occurred prior to the time that the children were speaking extensively." This generally accepted finding runs contrary to the long-held notion among psychologists that attributed the lack or inaccessibility of early memories to the young child's lack or tenuous grasp of language.

The capacity for retaining information about the past is evident in the everyday behavior of infants as well. The study of memory in infants, however, relies not on verbal responses about the past, but on the evidence of habituation, conditioning and other forms of learning. In a study with Dan Ashmead, Perlmutter relied upon parents trained to record in diaries the everyday use of memory in their seven, nine and eleven-month-old infants. "Albert eating lunch," reads one typical entry. "Handed Dorine [the babysitter] his glass. Dorine saw it was empty and filled it. He did the same for me several days ago. Twice during one meal he handed me his glass. Each time it was empty. Each time I filled it."

While all the infants in the study showed some spontaneous, or uncued, memory, such episodes were less frequent among the youngest infants. Perlmutter also found that older infants were actively involved in a greater percentage of memory episodes than younger infants. They were not just reacting to something remembered. "We think that this is evidence of something like recall memory beginning to appear in the older infants," she says.

Somewhere between the age of eight and twelve months a change does seem to occur in the infant's memory abilities.

Some psychologists perceive the nature of this change as a transition from recognition to recall memory, but others, such as Daniel Schacter and Morris Moscovitch of the University of Toronto, suggest that two different memory systems may be at work here. They refer to these systems as early and late memories. "The distinction," says Schacter, "is something along the line of implicit or procedural for the early memory, and explicit or declarative for the late memory."

To better understand the nature of this distinction, they used a simple task which Piaget made famous in 1954 to compare the mnemonic performance of amnesiacs and their degraded or impaired memory system with that of very young infants and their not-yet-fully-developed memory system. Piaget had observed that eight-to-ten-month-old infants can easily find an object when it is hidden at the same location (A) all the time. But after several successful searches at location A, many infants continue to search at A even though the infant has attended to the object's displacement into a different hiding place (B). Piaget called this phenomenon the AB Error.

"The amnesiac remembers where you put the object in the first place, just like the infant," Schacter says, "but then gets tripped up when you switch locations." But while the amnesiac, whose neurological state does not improve, continues to make the AB error, the infant stops making the error as he approaches his first birthday. To explain this improvement in performance, Schacter postulates the appearance of a late memory system. "We believe that the neural machinery that underlies the ability to remember the past may be in place within a year of birth, and that any further developments in memory are probably the result of building up the knowledge base and the integration of this machinery with other cognitive functions."

At the root of our attempt to understand how memory changes over time, and when autobiographical memory begins to develop, is perhaps the most intriguing question of all: What is the youngest age at which humans demonstrate memory? During the past decade studies of visual and auditory memory have shown that even the youngest of infants are consistently more responsive to novel stimuli than to familiar stimuli. These observations have led many psychologists to the conclusion that infants have a memory capacity from birth.

"Preverbal infants are able to encode and retain some information about their visual world from the first hours of life," notes Perlmutter. "Even neonates demonstrate this recognition memory." Others have extended this observation by demonstrating discrimination between novel and familiar stimuli in a group of premature infants with an average gestational age of thirty-five weeks.

Despite such evidence, psychologists have been rather reluctant to cross the birth barrier in order to trace the origins of memory. The area of pre-birth memory is a largely uncharted psychological territory. Even those who willingly concede that fetal memory is logically possible—that the fetus has the rudimentary capacity to encode experience—will cry foul at the claims for pre-birth memories.

"On one level the subject is very, very controversial," explains professor David Rubin, "but on another level it's totally dull. Why should the act of birth increase your learning abilities? Tony De Casper at the University of North Carolina at Greensboro found evidence for pre-birth memory by playing music to mothers in the hospital waiting to deliver. When their children were born they showed a preference for the music that had been played to them in utero. The study is very reputable. And we know that it could happen because the acoustics are there. There are studies in which microphones have been placed in the uterus of sheep and the sound is not muffled as much as you might think."

A controversial Toronto psychiatrist, Thomas Verny, believes that the first thin slivers of memory actually begin streaking across the fetal brain sometime during the third trimester. "To say that somehow children are radically different after birth from the way they were before birth simply doesn't make sense," says Verny. "The central nervous system does not change from one day to the next. By the age of six months after conception the neural circuits in the brain of the unborn child are just as advanced as they are in the newborn."

Verny's radical premise has largely been met with anger, criticism and scorn, except among those in the new field of pre and perinatal psychology. This discipline concerns itself with understanding the psychology of pregnancy and the ways in which the pregnant mother influences her unborn child's physical, intellectual and emotional development. Ernest Freud, the nephew of the founder of psychoanalysis, was among those speaking at the discipline's first international congress, held in Toronto in 1983.

"The best age to ask children about their memories is between two-and-a-half and three-and-a-half," Verny says, "after that they forget. Here, for instance is a conversation between a mother and her three-and-a-half-year-old." He picks up and reads one of the many letters he has received from parents since he wrote *The Secret Life of the Unborn Child* in 1981:

> I am putting away pictures to get ready for a move. Patton is helping me pack the empty frames and sees once again the picture of me hugely pregnant. 'Look how big your tummy is,' he says.
>
> Why is it so big? 'Because I was a baby and I was in there.'
>
> What was it like in there? 'There was a snake in there with me.'
>
> What was the snake doing in there with you? 'It was trying to eat me but it wasn't poisonous.'
>
> How did you get out of my tummy? 'I think it broke.'
>
> How did it break? 'I don't know.'
>
> What did you do when you got out of my tummy? 'I went to the hospital. And when your tummy broke I went to the hospital and that thing in my tummy broke out and got the snake out. The doggy said go away out of your tummy.'
>
> What doggy? 'There was a doggy in your tummy with me. I think it was Crystal. I think he was in your tummy with me.'
>
> What did you and Crystal do in my tummy? 'We played.'
>
> How? 'Like this (he waves his arms).'
>
> What did it sound like in my tummy? 'I don't know.'
>
> What color was it? 'I don't know.'
>
> Crystal is our dog whom we found as a puppy about five months before Patton was born. He spent much of the later part of my pregnancy on my stomach.

Few people consciously remember birth and pre-birth events, according to Verny, because of the oxytocin secreted by the mother during labor and birth. Oxytocin is the principal hormone for inducing uterine contractions and lactation, and studies have shown that the hormone induces amnesia in laboratory animals. Birth and pre-birth memories normally emerge only when psychiatrists and psychologists regress patients through drugs, hypnosis, free association and other means. "You can also find pre-birth memories in dreams," says Verny, "though most people are unaware that this is in fact what the dreams represent."

If the claims for birth and pre-birth memories are valid, then all the efforts being made to locate the beginnings of autobiographical memory in early childhood will be off the mark. But, in general, psychologists regard such claims with a good deal of suspicion and disbelief. They prefer to tread more traditional grounds for an answer to the question that led us through the maze of early memory in the first place: When does autobiographical memory begin to be established?

Katherine Nelson, a developmental psychologist at the City University of New York, has studied the question in connection with the scripts that children have for familiar events, and presents what is perhaps the most cogent hypothesis for the development of autobiographical memory. These "scripts" refer to the way children have organized their acquired knowledge in terms of general event structures. They would therefore have scripts for such familiar routines as eating dinner at home and going to the supermarket.

"There does seem to be a drive to build up these scripts," says Nelson. "It seems to come out of a biological need to understand what is going on, so the child doesn't need language or anything else, all he needs is the background of experience."

But in young children these scripts appear to block or override memories for specific experiences. Nelson found that children of three and four years of age, who can produce reasonably good general accounts of dinner at home, for example, have difficulties producing an account of a specific dinner. They will speak about "what happens" rather than "what happened." Perhaps this explains "why children insist upon the way things should be much more than adults," she says.

"It's possible that specific memories are lost as the child enters specific experiences into their more general scripts," Nelson says, "while unique events, like going to the circus, may be more memorable because they haven't been repeated. Many more of these details are held onto because they haven't been overridden by some further experiences. But after a while if you don't go to the circus, you will forget about it, because it's not adaptive to hold onto that memory if it's not going to tell you anything about the future. Why do we have memories if not for the purpose of being able to predict and control future happenings?"

"So one hypothesis that we have come up with," Nelson continues, "is that the establishment of an autobiographical memory depends upon the emergence of an event that is unique with respect to the scripts children have developed. This script building system appears by the age of one, probably earlier. Once the scripts have been built, things that then happen which are unique are added to memory as something new and novel. That happens at about the age of two or three."

By this age speech has also developed and memory begins to show signs of social construction. "We think that children are also taught to remember by their parents," Nelson says, "when they say such things as 'Do you remember when we went to the store last week and you said such and such?' So their memory becomes at least partially formulated in terms of language. At that point, at about the age of three, significant variations or events that are emotionally laden or salient in some other way begin to create a memory string that is uniquely human and social. That's when autobiographical memory begins."

While Nelson's view of early memory development does not pretend to explain the multitude of phenomena involved in memory, it certainly ties up many loose ends regarding autobiographical memory. If, as she says, memory proceeds from the accumulation of single novel experiences to scripts and then to unique events capable of being shared, then it should be easy to see why we, as adults, cannot remember specific autobiographical memories before about the fourth year of life. Such memories could not form until a significant general base of event knowledge had been established. And this, of course, would take a number of years to build up. Rome was not built in a day.

IMAGINARY COMPANIONS

We were all magicians once. Hidden away in the dusty attic of childhood memories lies a time when we stood astride two worlds. When we could erect fairy kingdoms with a few sticks or wooden blocks. When ferocious animals would spring from the shadows of our bedrooms at night. When the fire trucks and tractors we commandeered could sweep through the towering infernos and utopias of our imagination.

Then one day we gave up the notion that we could fly if given the chance, that trees and little girls in paintings could answer back when spoken to, that Santa Claus and the Easter Bunny were real. Gone, too, were those imaginary friends of ours like Scotty and Gink, who shared a seat at the dinner table with the family, took the blame for the naughty things we did, and were always around to play with, unlike most of the kids in the neighborhood.

But Stephen King, the modern master of the macabre, like some of us, still remembers his imaginary companion vividly. "I had one when I was six or seven," he says. "I was the younger of two boys. My brother was always off on his own. My mother worked, and I often hung around by myself. So I invented this kid to play with that nobody could see but me. His name was Jerry, and he hung around with me for two or three years. He was great. He did anything I wanted. If I had a deck of cards, Jerry would play war with me. If Jerry won, he would always be bighearted and magnanimous about it and never rub it in the way some of the other kids would."

Young children spend a good deal of their time in the world of make-believe and certainly the most common inhabitants of that realm are the extraordinary creations known as imaginary companions. These invisible characters, unlike other kinds of make-believe, often seem to occupy a physical space in the world of the child. "They have a reality which is very striking," says Dr. Humberto Nagera, a child analyst and professor of psychiatry at the University of Michigan Medical Center in Ann Arbor. "For the child, the imaginary companion has a presence that would not be possible at any other age."

A surprisingly large number of children have imaginary companions. They are very common, according to Dr. Jerome Singer, a professor of psychology at Yale University. He has spent much of his professional life studying fantasy in children. At some point in the first five or six years of life, from a third to a half of all children have imaginary playmates, he estimates.

Imaginary friends and other fantasies play an important role in the development of the growing child. They serve as constructive devices that allow young children to rehearse various roles and prepare for adult life. "Imaginary companions help children learn, experiment, deal with stress and master problems," says Nagera. "And, of course, they get a lot of pleasure out of them." For these reasons, the phenomenon of imaginary companions has been invaluable to researchers, providing insights into reactions to loneliness, problems of severe conscience, and the potential of the creative imagination.

Children who have imaginary companions are known to be clearly different from their more literal-minded peers. A study by Singer and two other Connecticut psychologists found children with imaginary companions to be less aggressive and less fearful than other children, and they seemed happier, too. Their language was also richer, and they showed greater concentration and cooperation. And despite the fact that they watched less television than other children, they were seldom bored.

The association between imaginary companions and creativity is perhaps even more significant. Some studies have shown that young people with genuine artistic talent report a greater frequency of imaginary companions and daydreams in childhood. "Imaginary companions turn out to be a good indicator of general imaginativeness," says Singer. The presence of an imaginary companion in childhood shows originality of thought, a tendency to seek novel experiences, and a focusing of the mind which remains unperturbed by contradiction and untouched by the dogmas and taboos of common sense.

Invisible playmates are a universal age-old phenomenon. "Guardian angels" assumed this role in more religious times, but these days children are more apt to adopt a television character like the Hulk or Superman for an imaginary friend. They begin to appear as early as the second year of life, when children enter a phase in which they are capable of symbolic or pretend play. The earliest make-believe friends usually take the form of animals; dogs predominate, but children will also report fantasy spiders, rats, even bears and lions.

The great majority of imaginary companions, however, are human characters about the same age and sex as their creators. Still, other children may prefer to ally themselves with exotic creatures or supernatural beings such as fairies, little people, or extraterrestrials. *The Journal of Genetic Psychology* reports that one young child began imagining entities called "House-kins." They were "horrible little creatures that ate our food and pinched people."

The animistic use of objects in this kind of dramatic play is not uncommon either. Take Natashia, for instance, then a two-year-old living in Charlottesville, Va. She was in the bathroom one day having an animated conversation, although she was alone. Danielle, her mother, walked in and asked who she was talking to. "It's my friend," Natashia replied. "Who is your friend?" her mother asked. Natashia pointed to the door and said: "The doorknob."

Nor is it uncommon for some children to have several imaginary companions, as Dr. Josephine Hilgard discovered during a Stanford University study of imaginary companions. She mentions an only child, Margaret, who overcame her loneliness by adopting an entire family, Mrs. McGullicuddy and her eight children. "They lived in my grandfather's pea patch," recalled Margaret while in college. "Mrs. McGullicuddy kept losing some of them and I had to help her find them. Sometimes the children came into the house and played with me." When Margaret's family moved, all of Mrs. McGullicuddy's family moved also.

Children usually become quite attached to their imaginary

playmates and some of them come to play a very active role in the household. And no wonder: Some of them can be heard and seen as vividly as if they were alive. Most of the time the playmate even has a distinct personality and appearance. Some are loyal and steadfast, others are naughty, an alter ego for their creators. Many talk a lot; nearly all are expert listeners.

Psychologists have discovered that each child's need determines what role such a companion will play. Loneliness is usually the reason a child creates an invisible playmate, although such children are not necessarily shy or withdrawn. They may simply need a substitute when human friends are absent. Children may also use imaginary friends to take the blame and avoid parental criticism for the trouble they get into. Some children project their hopes and fears through a fantasy friend, rather than confessing them as their own. Still other children endow their imaginary companions with all the attributes they lack so that the friend can participate in their parents' affection. At times, imaginary companions play a conscience or superego role, the way Jiminy Cricket did in Walt Disney's *Pinocchio.*

Most children abandon their imaginary companions by the time they enter school. Fantasies normally become internalized at this age. But there are cases in which such a playmate has lasted a decade or more, or appeared in the child's later years. They even appear in adults. In fact, the popular notion of invisible playmates rests almost entirely on the memorable 1950 movie *Harvey,* in which an adult, played by Jimmy Stewart, befriends an imaginary six-foot rabbit. To the other characters in the story, Stewart's bunny initially suggests drunkenness and hallucinations. Eventually, as the action draws to a close, Harvey is seen as a sign of health and happiness. The story, of course, is fictional, and in the real world adults who talk into thin air are usually seen as not-quite-right-in-the-head.

But Dr. Benjamin Spock, pediatrician to millions, tends to argue in the Harvey spirit. "I think everybody has imaginary companions, adults as well as children," he says. "It can happen at any stage of life, not that we believe in them as adults, of course. How much of our world is spent in make-believe varies enormously with the individual. After all, the novelist lives in a world of make-believe a good part of the time, certainly during the course of his writing. So does the actor and the playright."

Adults who speak to a fantasy are not necessarily crazy. "When someone feels a little lonely or in a strange place," says Singer, "they may imagine talking to someone who is important to them." The most common example is the wife or husband who is far away from home and imagines their spouse is present and talking.

But an imaginary companion encountered in an adult may also imply a psychopathological condition. Probably the most famous recent example can be found in the strange case of Mark David Chapman, John Lennon's killer. During proceedings that led to Chapman's sentencing, forensic psychiatrist Dr. Daniel Schwartz testified that from the age of about nine years Chapman had trouble socializing with other children. "Instead, he would spend much of his time alone," said Schwartz, "engrossed in an imaginary world. Initially it consisted of thousands of what he called 'little people' living in the walls of his living room."

"I had control over their lives," Chapman told Schwartz. "They would worship me like a king." And whenever the little people angered him, Chapman would wreak havoc by pressing an imaginary destruct button on the arm of his family sofa. Usually, however, their sovereign king was benign, and at times he would even stage imaginary concerts for his little people in which the Beatles would perform.

In time, Chapman's childhood kingdom became more democratic. He became the president, not a king, and his government consisted of a Senate and a House of Representatives, a variety of committees, and, most important, a cabinet to which he could turn for advice. Although the little people were no longer prominent in his life, they were not entirely forgotten. When Chapman began considering the murder of John Lennon in October, 1980, he consulted his cabinet. "They didn't want any part of it," Chapman later told Schwartz. "They were shocked."

There is indeed a dark side to this creative force. Despite the reassurances of child psychologists that imaginary companions are a sign of health, in a very few instances there is a basis for the fear that many educators and parents have expressed for generations: Could these creations be signs of incipient psychopathology?

"It depends on how exclusively the child is devoted to them," suggests Dr. Bruno Bettelheim, the world-renowned child psychologist, "whether they hamper or interfere with his adjustment to life. Like fantasies in general, within moderation, they are useful. In excess, they interfere. If a child lives entirely in a fantasy world and neglects reality, then we have some cause for concern. In adults, I would think, the situation would be more serious. The imaginary companions of deranged people are usualy persecutory figures and can become very active."

Many children will treat their invisible playmates as real, but most are well aware that their creations are pure fantasy, however loath they may be to admit the fact when questioned by adults. "What is most striking," says Nagera, "is that in spite of that knowledge they will still treat them as if they were real people."

How is this possible? It seems that for the child, the worlds of fantasy and reality exist side by side—they are not exclusive. Child's play appears to be a deliberate illusion, a refusal to allow the adult world to interfere with their play so that they may better enjoy that private reality. The late child psychologist Jean Piaget argued that the two-to-four-year-old child does not even question whether these symbolic creations are real or not. "He is aware in a sense that they are not so for others," wrote Piaget, "and makes no serious effort to persuade the adults that they are."

But parents and educators who believe that the child with an active fantasy life has a weak grasp on reality are mistaken. On the contrary, the child's contact with reality appears to be strengthened by those periodic excursions into fantasy. "Children with imaginary companions have a better idea of what is fact and what is fantasy than kids who don't have these imaginative resources," says Singer. "By exploring fantasy, the child learns to distinguish between fantasy and reality. Those who don't have much of a fantasy life might take the odd thought or particularly vivid image that comes into their minds as a real event."

While the normal child may quite easily distinguish between the two worlds, the disturbed child may not, and there, says Bettelheim, is the danger. "Many a child will play Superman," he says, "but only the troubled child will try to fly down from the third floor window. That's the difference between a fantasy that's healthy and one that's destructive."

A few psychologists even believe that there may be a link between imaginary companions and the experience of multiple personalities. "When we are kids," says Singer, "we make believe we are different kinds of people and have adventures for them in our mind's eye. Most people quickly dismiss these experiences, but others become very absorbed, engaging in a form of self-hypnosis in which they drift in and out of the other role without any real recollection.

"The multiple personality situation seems to start with an imaginary companion," he continues. "For whatever reason, the desire to identify with that person becomes so great, that they lose touch with reality and become absorbed with that other person, sometimes acting and talking like them. But this is an extremely rare phenomenon."

Once again, Chapman's story provides a classic example. In the fall of 1980, Chapman had begun to model himself after John Lennon, who like himself was married to a Japanese woman. "However, in a way peculiar to schizophrenics," said Schwartz, "the closer he came to achieving this goal of identifying with Mr. Lennon, the more he came to believing he was John Lennon." In fact, on his last day of work, October 23, he signed himself out as John Lennon. "I think what finally happened was this," Schwartz said. "Killing Mr. Lennon was, in his kind of schizophrenic reasoning, a compromise, a way of handling his own suicidal wishes, but in a sense, staying alive himself."

All of which has led some investigators to conclude that the line between the real and imaginary in these matters may sometimes be nonexistent. Some believe it may be a mistake to assume that all imaginary companions are figments of the child's imagination. "I've had a school teacher write to me from Connecticut saying that he's convinced they are real," says Singer. "He thinks they are real manifestations from the spirit world. Others have said the same thing to me, but I don't know what to make of it since I don't really believe in the spirit world." Could it be, though, that school teachers, being so close to so many children, might have an insight into the phenomenon that is not available to most lab-oriented researchers?

James Peterson, an elementary school teacher in Lafayette, California, whose masters thesis from the University of California, Berkeley, examined the subject of non-ordinary perception in children, insists on making a distinction between imaginary companions and invisible playmates. "An invisible playmate," he says, "is a kind of non-physical entity that is actually there objectively and isn't a figment of the child's imagination like the imaginary companion. It is something he is perceiving through some alternate mode of perception that is closed to us."

Often cited as an example that something quite apart from childhood imagination might be involved in these experiences is an account given by Louisa Rhine, the late noted psychic researcher. It involves a two-year-old boy whose parents rented a summer cottage at the New Jersey shore many years ago. Soon after their arrival, the mother heard her son, who had been napping in one of the bedrooms, say: "See man, see man." When she peeked into the room, she saw her son standing in the crib, smiling and pointing at nothing she could see. Sometimes he would offer his toys to the invisible man and urge his parents to come meet him.

At the end of their stay, the owner of the cottage dropped by to introduce herself. She explained that it was her first visit to the house since her husband had died there the previous year—in the very room used by the little boy. "He was so fond of children," the widow told the shocked parents.

Not all children with invisible companions are having paranormal experiences, says Peterson, but true invisible playmates are probably more common than is generally believed. The child's description of the invisible friend is usually enough to distinguish between the two. "If a child sees a twenty-five-foot brontosaurus that asks for bubble gum, I think it would be safe to say he is probably imagining it," he explains. "But if a young child begins to have long discussions with an older man about the nature of God and the possibility of life after death, then it might be well to investigate the possibility that the paranormal is involved."

That some imaginary companions may actually be denizens from some nether world is certainly an intriguing notion. But just as intriguing is the human capacity for imagination. That a young child can plunge into the world of fantasy in search of a solution that satisfies some inner need, only to re-emerge into the real world with a phantom friend in hand, is a Herculean feat of creativity. Says Singer: "The development of a fantasy friend may be one of the first great creative acts of the growing child."

INNER SELVES

"Things are getting very secretive here now. Mr. Kugler was afraid that they might come here to search for hidden bicycles and for that reason he wanted to have the door leading to our place camouflaged. They have done that now in such a way that it looks like a wall cabinet with books."—Anne Frank, Aug. 21, 1942.

The Diary of Anne Frank is perhaps this century's most celebrated evocation of the interior life. It was begun when Anne was thirteen, just before she, her family and friends went into hiding from the Nazis in a small apartment in the city of Amsterdam, and ended shortly after her fifteenth birthday, when the Nazis raided their hideout.

Anne Frank's moving story stands out as one of the finest examples of diary as literature. Most diaries, however, fail as literature for one simple reason—they are boring. They are cluttered with faceless characters, endless dinner menus, postcard sceneries, and dreary household trivia. Worse still, they are repetitious. One diarist faithfully recorded his daily routine—getting up, eating, reading and praying—more than three thousand times in his diary. "The journal is a record of experiences and growth," noted Henry David Thoreau, "not a preserve of things well done or said."

Looked at in this way, the practice of keeping a journal becomes a task of considerable psychological significance. "When you take into account the number of diaries that are being written today," says Sharyn Lowenstein, the author of a dissertation for Boston University entitled "The Journal Journal-Keeper Relationship," "diary keeping can be seen as an important phenomenon in its own right."

By every conceivable measure, journal writing seems a very popular activity, despite the effects of the telephone on the ancient practice of putting the pen to paper. Some ten thousand diaries and journals have been published in the English language alone and hundreds more are added to the shelves each year. Tens of thousands of people across the country have participated in the popular journal-writing workshops offered by the psychologist Ira Progoff. But the most telling statistic comes from diary manufacturers, who estimate that more than five million blank books or empty diaries are sold each year. And while these traditional "Dear Diaries" are still widely used, more and more people have been turning to alternative journal formats—to rapid ones such as tape recorders, and to easily accessible ones such as spiral-bound notebooks, yellow legal pads, and scraps of paper scribbled on and stuffed into a drawer or shoebox.

The practice is so prevalent that diaries can often be found in the shadows of many a news event. At least three of the American hostages kept diaries during their 444 days of captivity in Iran, but only one, Sgt. Rodney "Rocky" Sickmann, managed to smuggle his out. President Harry Truman preserved his thoughts in a journal format in which he revealed his difficulties with Gen. Douglas MacArthur, whom he called "Mr. Prima Donna." Jimmy Carter also kept a diary during his presidency, as did Dwight Eisenhower; Richard Nixon kept his on tape. The psychotic killer, David Berkowitz, known as "Son of Sam," also kept a diary, in which he wrote: "There is no doubt in my mind that a demon has been living in me since birth." Baring her soul—and more—in an issue of *Playboy,* Rita Jenrette, the ex-wife of the former South Carolina Representative who was convicted during the Abscam scandal, told a reporter that she had kept a diary for years.

"Why do I feel compelled to write down all these little ideas and notions?"—Saxon Holt, Jan. 9, 1981.

There appear to be almost as many reasons for keeping a journal as there are journal keepers. "It's a habit, just like orange juice in the morning," says Bliem Kern, an astrologer and poet in New York. "I do it for the simple pleasure of writing," says Craig Schenck, a bartender in New Orleans. "I keep a journal as a testimony to the fact that I have lived, not just existed," says James Cummings. "I think there is a hell of a difference." Cummings is an antiquarian-book dealer and collector in Stillwater, Minnesota, whose old Victorian home houses the largest collection of diaries in the world—more than ten thousand volumes.

Children who were once encouraged to keep a diary either by a teacher or through the gift of a blank book may also continue the practice out of habit. Those in the midst of celebrated people may feel the itch to record, as may the soldier in the chaos of war. Traveling seems to bring out the writer in nearly everyone. Politicians, entertainers and other public figures may keep a journal if they are concerned about what the historical record will have to say about them. Writers often mention that journal keeping provides them with subject matter and helps them develop a natural style.

But most often, journal writing is cited by practitioners for its cathartic function. The journal is, and has been throughout history, a tool for self-understanding. "It's really a release for me," says a photographer in San Francisco. A graphic artist in Washington, D.C. says: "It's a good way of keeping track of yourself and then looking back to find out how you survived."

The journal is not a perfect instrument, however. It can create problems as well as solve them. The author Henry Miller believed that the problem with journal writing was one of arithmetic. "You will never catch up with the days," he once told Anaïs Nin, a prolific diarist whose work has had a profound influence on twentieth-century journal keeping. "It will be like a big web which will strangle you."

For the most part, diary keeping is a closet practice, and most of its practitioners are unaware that they are part of a long cultural and historical tradition. Some observers trace journal writing back to cave paintings, but others believe it did not begin until much later. "The idea of writing down daily thoughts and notes on passing events, especially when it takes a more or less introspective form, is of comparatively modern growth," Ponsonby wrote in his first volume of *English Diaries.*

The first diaries of a consistently introspective nature were written by ladies of the royal Japanese court in the tenth century. These records took the form of pillow books, so called because they were tucked in or under the pillow. Their diaries probed beyond the historical surface of life and extended the written record of daily experience to include inner realms as well—dreams, fantasies, even fiction. One entry, from the diary of Murasaki Shikibu, a lady of the royal court in the first decade of the tenth century, has been the inspiration for many Japanese artists in their paintings:

"I wish I could be more adaptable and live more gaily in the present world—had I not an extraordinary sorrow—but whenever I hear delightful or interesting things, my yearning for a religious life grows stronger. I become melancholy and lament. I try to forget, for sorrow is vain. Am I too sinful? So I was musing one morning when I saw waterfowl playing heedlessly in the pond."

The practice of diary writing blossomed in the West during the Renaissance. But Samuel Pepys, who was born in 1633, is regarded by many critics as the Shakespeare of diarists. He found in the diary a place to confess to God and account for his life. It was also a natural place, Pepys and other gentlemen of the time discovered, to record travel experiences. A journey was, to them, a perfect analogy to life.

With effortless frankness, utmost confidence and great humor, Pepys treated his inner and outer lives with equal respect—and demonstrated what a diarist can do at his literary best. Here is a portion of his entry for Oct. 13, 1660:

"I went out to Charing Cross, to see Major General Harrison hanged, drawn and quartered; which was done there, he looked as cheerful as any man could do in that condition. He was presently cut down, and his head and heart shown to the people, at which there was great shouts of joy. . . .From thence to my Lord's, and took Captain Cuttance and Mr. Shebly to the Sun Tavern, and did give them some oysters. After that I went by water home, where I was angry with my wife for her things lying about, and in my passion kicked the little fine basket, which I bought her in Holland, and broke it, which troubled me after I had done it."

Thirteen years before Pepys's birth, the diary had arrived in America on the Mayflower with the Puritans, who may have been the most prolific diarists of all time. Their diaries, which greatly influenced the development of the modern diary, were kept as a hedge against despair and were based on the belief that salvation could be attained through self-examination. The Quakers, too, kept diaries as a way of making their lives witnesses to God.

Diaries gradually became less a spiritual tool and travalogue and more an instrument of release as Europeans began rebelling against a ruling class that ignored their individuality. The intensely introspective form of the diary that arose at about the time of the French Revolution was known as the *journal intime.* The *journal intime* became an excruciatingly detailed examination of the conscience and the emotions. Stendhal, who began his journal at the age of eighteen, captured the mercurial responsiveness that is the essence of the *journal intime* in his entry for Sept. 11, 1811: "I note the echo that each thing produces as it strikes my soul."

The journal traveled westward in the United States when hundreds of pioneer women created a network of correspondence and mutual support that was based on a shared interest in journal writing. "In fact, so many women relied on the diary to preserve their history and culture," writes Tristine Rainer, in *The New Diary,* "that two hundred years later, many people had come to think of the diary as primarily a woman's mode of expression."

The exploration of the woman's experience in the diaries of Anaïs Nin, first published in 1966, had a considerable impact on the women's movement and on the number of women who began keeping diaries. "She emphasized the importance of women's articulateness at this time in history and demonstrated how the diary could help them find their own expressive language," writes Rainer, a co-founder of the women's studies programs at the University of California, Los Angeles. Women from all over the world identified with Anaïs Nin's diaries. They wrote her letters saying, "It's like my diary."

*"Bypass this weekend, avoid it, draw a line. . .from Friday to
Sunday night, wrap it, like a bale of cotton, throw it over-
board."*—Colette Nivelle, summer, 1978.

The diary is, first and foremost, a psychological tool, an instrument for self-understanding. Those who recognize it as
such look upon their diaries as companions and confidants.
Like a good therapist, the diary is the perfect listener. In fact,
the word "therapist" in its original Greek form, *theraput,*
means "attendant."

The services of the attendant are normally required during
times of stress. "The life of a diary is often born of a tension, a
disequilibrium in the life of its author, which needs to be solved
or held in check," writes Steven Kagle in *American Diary Literature.* People in a crisis will write. Not surprisingly, many journal keepers begin their personal jottings during adolescence, a
time when the young person becomes conscious of his unique-
ness and solitude and may feel that adults can no longer fathom
his needs. In later life, diaries are frequently attempts to fend
off a different sort of chaos, to bring order, coherence and purpose to one's subjective world.

Therapists of many different theoretical approaches have
come to recommend the journal in therapy because of its useful-
ness as a self-monitoring technique. Behavioral therapists urge
their patients to keep a record of their behavior with regard to
a specific problem, such as obesity, depression or cigarette
smoking. "It's a very goal-oriented approach," says Dr. Albert
Stunkard, a professor of psychiatry well known for his work on
obesity and weight control at the University of Pennsylvania.
"What we try to do is focus in on the person's problem, which,
in the case of obesity, may be how often the patient eats during
the day, when he eats, what he eats, whom he eats with or what
his mood is when he eats. Once you've narrowed it down, you
simply have the patient keep count of the problem behavior.
This self-monitoring technique is very reinforcing for the patient."

Many cognitive therapists also use the journal in therapy.
"We use journals to find out what people are telling themselves," says Albert Ellis, a psychotherapist and the founder of
the Institute for Rational-Emotive Therapy in New York. Jour-

nals, says Ellis, help people identify and correct the irrational and unrealistic thought patterns that are at the root of depression and many other problems.

Jungian analysts also advocate the use of the journal as a therapeutic tool, primarily to record dreams. "We use the journal as a way of recording the individual's deeper experiences over time," says June Singer, a California psychotherapist and interpreter of Jungian thought in such books as *Boundaries of the Soul.* "The journal gives you a sense of a journey that the analysis really is."

Therapists realize that the diary is a natural outgrowth of the clinical situation, in which the patient is usually encouraged to speak for himself. "I think one of the very important things about journal keeping in therapy is that it takes the responsibility of the process out of just that hour or two a week," says Singer. "Journal keeping commits the individual to develop a psychological attitude, to recognize that whatever we see is based on our own experience, based on what we have tapped into from our ancestral pool, based on our interaction with the environment, all of which makes each individual's view of reality unique. We really find out who we are through journals."

"I no longer want him. I hate myself. I hate D. He is stupid and too rough tonight. He hurts me. I cannot understand why I don't enjoy him. I don't even feel comfort in his warmth."—Sheri Russell, March 21, 1974.

Journal writing is a ritual by which individuals struggle to understand themselves and their most intimate relationships, according to Barbara Myerhoff, a professor of anthropology at the University of Southern California, and Deena Metzger, a poet and creative-writing instructor in Los Angeles. They believe that the journal performs the task assigned to it by the psyche in three stages. The first stage, differentiation, begins with putting the words on the page, which allows the individual to behold the inner self, just as the mirror allows a view of the outer self.

In the second stage, the self is then free to contemplate itself in all its manifestations. It is here that feelings of loneliness, weakness and doubt are recorded, private feelings that cannot be communicated even to the closest friends. It is here that the diarist can freely admit what the California researchers call "the beasts and monsters, imaginings and wishes, lies and fantasies," while at the same time holding at bay "the tyranny of public interpretation."

The diarist will often keep the work a secret, thus preventing embarrassing revelations from coming to light and allowing the emerging self to be its own first witness. Particularly troublesome material may be transformed into poetry, short stories or paintings. And to insure further secrecy, the diarist may utilize a multitude of ingenious strategies, from locking the journal in a desk drawer or hiding it on a closet shelf among the linens to camouflaging it in foreign languages, codes or shorthand. Pepys wrote in a shorthand made even more difficult by ciphers of his own invention and phrases in bastardized Latin and French.

In the final stage of the process, the journal writer reviews the outpouring and integrates and reincorporates the newly uncovered material. At this point, a quantum jump in understanding may occur. "When we go deeply into the personal," says Anaïs Nin, "we go beyond the personal. We achieve something that is collective."

In certain situations, the journal can be a hazardous instrument. For some people, says Albert Ellis, "it can do more harm than good." The journal can lock people in circular attitudes and behaviors. One diarist describes the feeling as "being trapped in a house of mirrors." Henry Fynes Clinton, a nineteenth-century journal keeper noted: "Many minor problems are magnified in importance by being registered in the journal, and a morbid sensibility generated." And often, the diarist, while mulling over emotions, may not think to record the basic elements of security and happiness that knit life to family and friends. "Once after reading my diary," says one New York diarist, surprised at the gloomy content of her writing, "I remember making a note to myself: 'I am not depressed all the time.'"

Not all journal keepers successfully manage to use the journal as a tool to understand themselves better. Some simply fail to reread their diaries. "And the journal does not reach the depth it can unless it gets started in the therapeutic process," says therapist Singer, though she concedes that many individuals "get a lot out of journal writing without therapy." The success of the journal seems to depend a great deal on the individual keeping it.

That knowledge has led Ira Progoff, a New York City psychologist who is best known for his work on journal keeping, to be highly critical of ordinary diaries. "The charge is usually made of journal keeping that it leads to subjectivity and solipsism, and I think that it's true," says Progoff. "It's the side of the culture that becomes narcissistic and subjectively self-concerned that goes in for diary keeping."

Progoff views most journal keeping as a fad. People will often start a diary during troubled times only to put it down when the situation improves. Journals don't solve any problems, he says. "Freudian analysts over the years have opposed journal keeping. They feel that you get rid of emotion without solving the problem. I think they are correct. The diary keeper may feel better for a while, but it's misleading. It's like taking a pain killer for a bad toothache—and later the abscess explodes."

Most journals are inadequate, he says, because they are static tools. They are used not so much as an instrument for growth as for self-justification. "I fear one lies more to one's self than to anyone else," Lord Byron wrote in his diary. Progoff agrees, adding that many individuals use a journal to insulate themselves against questions they do not wish to face. Louis XVI may have fallen into that trap. On the day the Bastille was stormed, he entered in his diary a single word: "Nothing."

Just how effective the journal can be as a psychological tool depends entirely upon the person using it. Only the person with a strong creative flair can unlock the journal's potent powers, says Progoff—people like Anaïs Nin, for example. But most people have no ropes to hold onto, have no structure to guide them in keeping a journal and, as a result, have no way of breaking through the circular attitudes and behaviors that journal keeping fosters.

To avoid these limitations, Progoff developed his own system of journal writing, a structured psychological workbook which he calls The Intensive Journal. The idea germinated back in the 1960s while he was director of the Institute for Research in Depth Psychology at Drew University in New Jersey. By studying the lives of creative people like Fyodor Dostoyevsky and Samuel Taylor Coleridge, Progoff found that creative people were much more aware of and attuned to their lives than were noncreative people. So Progoff developed a set of procedures to be applied in a journal format that would evoke the underlying process of growth that seemed to him to occur in the lives of these creative people.

The keeper of an Intensive Journal gathers data in a large, loose-leaf notebook divided into nearly two dozen subsections. There is a "Dream Log," a "Twilight Imagery Log," a "Steppingstones" section, and there are sections for "Dialogues" with persons, events, work and the body. Material for these sections emerges through reflection, free association, imagery, meditation, recollection, and spiritual exercise. The sections "feedback" on one another, according to Progoff, and aid the individual in integrating the relationships among the various people, events and ideas in one's life. It is an instrument, he says, for finding the inner connecting thread, or meaning, in our lives.

Ira Progoff has organized thousands of Intensive Journal workshops across the country through the Dialogue House in New York City. The workshops cost under one hundred dollars, and most participants, though not all, say the method works. Others have learned it on their own through Progoff's book, *At a Journal Workshop.* No doubt, part of his success stems from the fact that, as one diary afficionado put it, "people are so accustomed to have somebody help them get started in something." In any case, his promotion of the Intensive Journal method has contributed a great deal to the current growth in journal writing in general.

"I throw away my diaries a few weeks after they are completed. They are like millstones around my neck. I don't like being encumbered by the past."—Craig Schenck.

The destruction of journals is a common experience among

diary keepers and, occasionally, a very useful one. "I've had many patients who do that," says Ira Progoff. "I remember saying to one young woman, 'Better your journal than you.' It's the identification of oneself with the journal. When a diarist does this, it's a kind of symbolic suicide. I always think that when people try to commit suicide they are not trying to kill themselves—they are just trying to get rid of the past. But sometimes they are clumsy."

Whether saved to be reread or destroyed to liberate its writer from the past, the diary is, at the very least, a comforting instrument, a home for private terrors and bafflements. Using it to its full potential, however, the diary keeper may find diary and life constantly feeding off one another. "There is an incentive to make your life interesting," said Anaïs Nin, "so that your diary will not be dull."

The diary—an odd, curiously sensitive device, immensely powerful in the hands of the gifted person—takes on a life of its own. "Usually," wrote E.B. White, an inveterate journal keeper, "when a man quits writing in his journal. . .he has lost interest in life."

GROUP DREAMING

"Dreams belong to dreamers," says Chris Hudson, a former apple orchard worker, describing the concept behind his effort to encourage dream communities across the country. "There are no experts in dreaming except for the dreamers themselves." So far his newsletter, the *Dream Network Bulletin,* has linked up about two thousand individuals, some of whom live as far away as Yugoslavia and Australia. What they all have in common is an interest in sharing their dreams and using them, when possible, to help one another.

Today there are dream communities all across the country. New Jersey has a dream community, as do California, Colorado, Kansas, Michigan, Massachusetts, Maine, Florida, and Puerto Rico. Their size and popularity vary. Those in the New York City area who are involved in the dream-community concept, for example, are about three hundred strong. These communities are where the people's dreams and accompanying visions, yearnings and hopes, come to the surface. Participants say that it's here, where two or more people get together to talk about dreams, that the magic happens.

The idea of establishing such communities of dreamers began in the early 1970s. Henry Reed started it all. "It's true," says Reed, a frizzy-haired, blue-eyed dream scientist who lives in a modest lakefront home in Virginia Beach, Virginia. "I was probably the originator of the group-dreaming experiment in modern culture. But all I did really was bring up-to-date a tradition that is long-standing, especially among American Indians."

Reed's story is that of a modern-day shaman. He was afflicted. He was cured. He made his cure available to others. His affliction, Reed admits openly, was alcoholism. The cure came as the result of a graphic dream in which he saw the image of a wine bottle coupled with a repulsive image of oozing, suppurating sores. The imagery of the dream was so potent, it became the catalyst that set him on the road to recovery.

His idea for a dream community also came, appropriately, from a dream. He and a group of associates were wandering in the dark, but when they started dancing in a strange, ceremonial way, the dark dreamscape exploded into light. Later on, after speaking of this dream in a talk, Reed was told it closely resembled the sun dance, a religious ceremony of the Plains Indians. Reed liked the title, and in the mid-1970s he began putting out a publication, the *Sundance Community Dream Journal,* to encourage those interested in the phenomenon of dreaming to come together and share their experiences and visions.

"I was trying to create an alternative scientific community that anyone could participate in by virtue of his being a dreamer," he explains, "because in effect every dreamer is a researcher, and every dream is an experiment in consciousness."

His role as a shaman came into being when he thought there might be some therapeutic potential in dreams. Reed, who is a licensed professional counselor, was experimenting with a process whereby certain individuals would spend three days meditating on a problem, making a conscious effort to dream about it, in order to arrive at some new insights.

"Part of the philosophy of the dream-incubation procedure," explains Reed, "is to encourage the dreamer to share the benefits of the dream quest with the rest of the community." But when Reed began conducting the dream-incubation procedure in group or community settings, something quite unexpected happened. The person incubating a dream often got "spied" on in the dreams of the other members of the community. Some people, in other words, found themselves dreaming about that person's problem even without having been told what it was. This has become known as group dreaming.

Reed talked about this phenomenon with clinical psychologist Robet Van de Castle, a professor in the Department of Behavioral Medicine at the University of Virginia Medical School and director of the Nocturnal Cognition Laboratory, the university's dream laboratory. Van de Castle himself had been a subject in dream-telepathy experiments back in the 1960s and had a long-standing interest in the subject. Together, Van de Castle and Reed decided to try to tap into this dream resource.

Out of their efforts came something called the dream-helper experiment. In it, a group of people are asked to concentrate their dreaming on an individual and his problem, which is never stated. The day before the dream night, some of the dreamers may meditate with the person or just spend time with him. The following morning, when the group members gather to recount their dreams, they are often surprised to find they have shared dreams with similar details. Reed and Van de Castle call these individuals dream helpers.

"Each would pick up a piece of a puzzle," Van de Castle says of their special dreams. "It's a little like the blind men with an elephant. When they put the pieces together they had the whole picture." After each dream helper reports what he dreamed, the target person, whose problem was the subject of the dream, is encouraged by Reed and Van de Castle to discuss the images as they might relate to the problem. Very often some valuable insight comes of the session.

When dreaming about one woman's problem, for example, the group shared a recurring image of water. It turned out the woman had a phobia of water. Discussing the various dream images with the group helped her focus on how that phobia came about and gave her the courage to consider learning how to swim again.

In another instance, an enigmatic but apparently harmless dream of objects helped break down the reserve of one of the target persons in a Van de Castle experiment. She was a shy woman who was not at all forthcoming in seeking help. But one of the helper's dreams, in which he saw objects whizzing through the air as if by their own volition, triggered a powerful reaction in her. As it happened, she was brooding over her unhappy childhood. Her mother had died when she was a small child, and her father had remarried. The stepmother and her two children disliked the girl and tormented her. A favorite daily cruelty of her stepbrother and stepsister was to throw stones at her as she walked home from school. The dream brought back that memory and precipitated the emotional breakthrough that caused her to seek help.

Because it seemed to uncover unspoken thoughts, the dream-helper experiment smacked of telepathy and seemed to confirm a long-held notion among psi (ie., ESP and psychokinesis) researchers that telepathy was more likely to occur when put to some practical use rather than when tested solely for the sake of a lab experiment. It seemed that by comparing the dreams of the collective, one could determine the telepathic content and study how telepathy gets disguised in dream material. Even more significant, dream-helper telepathy seemed to be replicable; you could get it to recur.

Initially Reed was excited about this aspect of his discovery. He thought he had a way of testing psi. But he quickly realized that the test was a less-than-perfect tool for psi research. To begin with, the target person's problem is often multifaceted, not easy to summarize in a single image or dream. In addition, the process of relating the helpers' dreams to the target can be done only with the help of the target himself, a subjective process that is more art than science.

As an example of the layers a problem might have, Reed tells the story of one young woman who had difficulty, she thought, choosing what college to transfer to and what area of study to pursue. But when the group went to dream about this, many reported confusing imageries that had nothing to do with school but instead seemed to be related to illicit sex. It turned out that the woman had had an affair with a married man. When the group told her of their dreams, she realized that it was not just a question of choosing a school and a subject but of deciding whether to stay with her lover. With the group's help she decided to move and ended up pursuing a successful career.

Of course, the dream-helper phenomenon may well occur quite naturally and unconsciously in everyday life. And if it does, if dreams do indeed peek outside the world of the dreamer and provide valid, verifiable information about the world, then it seems that such knowledge could be put to good use in other areas.

Researchers at the University of Cape Town, in South Africa, think so. They have found that interpreting a collection of a family's dreams can be almost as informative as the kind of diagnostic information a family therapist gleans from personal interviews. In one experiment, five families were asked to keep dream diaries and also to go to a family therapist. Each family member was interviewed by a therapist who didn't see the diaries. And each dream diary was examined by a dream interpreter who didn't meet the individuals. The experiment found that in 70 percent of the cases, the dream interpreter agreed with the interviewing therapist's assessments of the families' problems. At times dream interpretation even provided additional information that had been undetected by the family therapist.

But the value of the group-dreaming concept has implications far beyond therapy. "There may be political ramifications to the process of a group of people focusing their dreams on a central topic," says Reed. "We know that the unconscious shapes society. If we can become aware of this process, we can nurture it and foster its growth into some visible and practical consequence."

SPEECHLESS

If feelings are the basic currency of human emotions, then some of us have been shortchanged. Take the case of the engineer whose history of intractable headaches thwarted his lifelong ambition to become an airline pilot. When asked how he felt about the situation, he replied: "I don't know what you expect me to say when you ask how I feel." Or take the case of the woman who, when asked how she felt about her mother's death, replied: "Well, it wasn't good. But the flowers were pretty."

That some people lack the vocabulary necessary to express their feelings is a well-established medical fact. The condition, which might be a harmless trait for some people but a severe problem for others, is known to psychiatrists as *alexithymia*, a term that means *without words for feelings*. Psychiatrists estimate that more than ten percent of the population may be alexithymic.

Alexithymics are typically described as emotional illiterates. They have very little awareness of their emotional lives and normally cannot distinguish between even such common emotions as sadness and anxiety. Their thinking is preoccupied with the minutiae of external events and they lead bleak fantasy lives. Most deny that they ever dream.

"The problem is that these people cannot connect their thoughts with their emotions," says Dr. Peter Sifneos, the Harvard professor of psychiatry who coined the term alexithymia.

"Emotions are not the same thing as feelings," he explains, "though dictionaries often don't differentiate between the two. Emotions are biological. A cat can have an emotion when it sees a dog coming at it. But the cat can't have thoughts in reference to the situation. That's something we have that the cat doesn't. So we have feelings, namely the thoughts that are attached to the emotions. Alexithymics don't have that."

The condition has been observed in hypochondriacs, drug addicts, alcoholics, sociopaths, people with psychosomatic illnesses, and people who have experienced severe traumas. But alexithymia may also appear in people who are otherwise considered to be quite normal.

"I would say there are quite a lot of alexithymic individuals around," says Sifneos, "though most of them are unaware of having a problem at all. These people can function quite adequately, particularly in a technological and materialistic society such as ours. They can be creative and intelligent and make a lot of money. It's only when it comes to dealing with feelings and emotions that they have a problem. If one alexithymic marries another, they might have a wonderful marriage. But if an alexithymic husband has a neurotic wife, for instance, then all hell breaks loose."

Though alexithymia is a new word, it is not a novel idea. Sifneos himself began to describe the condition almost a decade before he coined the term, in 1972. He first came across such individuals during his work on dynamic short-term psychotherapy, a very active, conflict-oriented form of treatment that Sifneos pioneered in this country. Sifneos discovered that some of his patients didn't do well with this therapy because they were unable to describe how they felt. He noticed that many of these people also seemed to have psychosomatic problems.

Sifneos began to wonder if psychosomatic illnesses—from ulcerative colitis to eczema and rheumatoid arthritis—might not be by-products of the alexithymic personality. Instead of letting off emotional pressures and tensions by talking about them the way most of us do, alexithymics might be releasing their emotions through somatic channels.

But the situation may not be quite so simple, according to Dr. Charles Ford, a professor of psychiatry at the Vanderbilt University Medical Center, in Nashville, Tennessee, and the author of the book *The Somatizing Disorders*. "Alexithymia alone may not be enough to explain the appearance of psychosomatic illness," he suggests. "I suspect that these people come from fairly emotionally restricted backgrounds and lower socioeconomic classes and have been under higher levels of stress all of their lives."

Ford finds the concept of alexithymia quite valuable and useful nonetheless. "I think it is a very important concept," he says, "and we use it a great deal because it has profound implications for what kind of treatment you might suggest for patients."

Alexithymia makes quite clear that the psychoanalytic approach is not always the best form of treatment, especially for people who are incapable of expressing their emotions in words. Psychoanalysis only tends to make alexithymics more anxious. Sifneos recommends medication, behavior modification techniques, or group therapy.

Ford favors group therapy himself. "That can help improve the situation," he says, "but it won't turn an alexithymic into the kind of sensitive, emotional, empathetic—and sometimes neurotic—individual that many of us tend to be. Life is relatively simple for many of these people, and if the condition is not causing them any distress, I would not recommend any treatment at all."

Alexithymia has proved to be an attractive concept among psychiatrists, and as a result there has been no dearth of theories to explain the causes that underlie the condition. Sociocultural explanations stress the correlation with lower socioeconomic class and lack of social learning; psychoanalytic theories emphasize early developmental difficulties where mother-child interactions have been disrupted so that the child has not learned to describe his feelings. Studies of twins indicate that the condition may also have some genetic component.

But the most promising of all theories come from neurophysiology. It seems that many alexithymic characteristics can be understood as an interruption of communication between the brain's two hemispheres. Lending much support to this hypothesis are studies conducted on split-brain patients by UCLA clinical psychiatrist Dr. Klaus Hoppe and his colleagues.

Split-brain patients are those who have undergone a commissurotomy, an operation in which the brain's right hemisphere is severed from the left hemisphere. In right-handed people, the right hemisphere tends to be important in generating and interpreting emotions, while the left hemisphere seems to be more involved in verbal expression.

Hoppe's latest study indicates that people who have undergone commissurotomies show a much higher degree of alexithymia than those from similar socioeconomic background who have not had the operation. This suggests to Hoppe that people who are naturally alexithymic may be functionally commissurotomized, that is, they tend to have weak connections between their two brain halves.

Despite these insights, many questions still need to be answered. It is not known, for example, whether alexithymics can recognize their emotions but simply cannot express them verbally, or whether they cannot even recognize their emotions at all. "I think these people have emotions but that they can neither recognize nor express them," says Ford. "Of course, if they can't express them, it is very difficult to know whether they can recognize them or not. That's the Catch-22."

THE AWARENESS FACTOR

"Oh my god," says one member of the surgical team, looking down at the obese woman under deep anesthesia. "They dragged up another beached whale into our operating room." The jokes fly fast for the moment, but later the woman's very poor recovery will be no laughing matter. A week after surgery she will spontaneously remember the incident, and within twenty-four hours her mysterious surgical problem will have cleared up. Noticing the change, her nurse will check with someone who had been present at the operation and confirm that the insult had in fact taken place.

This true story is typical of reports known to physicians as "awareness under anesthesia." Their use of the term actually covers a broad spectrum of reports. At one extreme are patients who were inadequately anesthetized and who did in fact wake up in the middle of an operation. At the other end of the spectrum are fully anesthetized patients who have no conscious memory of their surgery but whose later behavior indicate a knowledge of events under anesthesia.

Most patients will remember nothing of their operation. "Only about one percent of all anesthetized patients experience some recall, with or without pain, of events during surgery," estimates Dr. Jacob Mainzer, an anesthesiologist at the University of New Mexico. "The basic problem is that the patients weren't given enough anesthesia. Like the trend toward lite beer, there is now also a trend toward lighter anesthetics." Modern anesthesiology uses more narcotics and muscle relaxants in order to use less anesthesia which, he explains, "is hard on the heart."

42

But the real issue behind these so-called episodes of awareness under anesthesia actually has very little to do with memory retrieval. The real story concerns whether or not perception
and memory formation is possible under anesthesia, and
whether or not consciousness is a prerequisite for awareness.
The first and most basic question to be answered is: Can perception occur in this unconscious state? In other words, does the
patient's nervous system continue to process the environment
under anesthesia?

"There is no reason to believe that perception is not functioning for meaningful information," says Henry Bennett, a psychologist on the faculty of the Department of Anesthesiology at
the University of California Davis Medical Center in Sac-
ramento. "General anesthetics do not turn off the entire nervous system during surgery. The sites where anesthetics have
their main effect are not those which control sensory integration. It is, in fact, fairly well known by people who are interested in the nervous system that the auditory system, for instance, is remarkably resistant to the effects of anesthetic
agents."

The idea that cognitive functioning is an ongoing process
even during unconsciousness has found new support in recent
experimental research with animals. A team of psychobi-
ologists—consisting of Norman Weinberger and Debra
Sternberg of the University of California at Irvine and Paul
Gold at the University of Virginia—managed to have anesthetized rats learn to fear a noise by injecting them with
epinephrine, a hormone which is thought to play an important
role in memory storage.

The rats were placed under heavy anesthesia and then presented with a series of tones followed by shocks. Some of the
rats were given epinephrine, while others received a saline solution. A week later the rats' reaction to the tones was tested
during a water drinking task. Those rats which had been injected with the saline solution continued to drink while those
which had received the epinephrine went off into a corner and
hid.

The experiment indicates that memories can form under
anesthesia, and helps explain some episodes of human awareness under anesthesia. "Since we know that epinephrine levels

rise in response to stress," says Gold, "it is my guess that those patients who do remember things that went on during surgery are those who reacted to the onset of their operation with this sort of hormonal response."

Studies of the rat's psychological cousin, the human being, support the notion that we are open to suggestion while anesthetized. In one study, the psychologist Henry Bennett played a tape to anesthetized patients asking them to touch their ears in a post-operative interview to indicate having heard the message. Nine of eleven patients later responded to the ear pulling suggestion. In another study, Bennett had patients under surgery successfully raise the temperature in one hand and lower the temperature in the other when asked to do so.

"We showed that patients under anesthesia are responsive to suggestion," says Bennett. "They can act on the suggestion after surgery *even though they could not consciously recall it.*" The medical consequence of such a "conscious unconscious," or "unconscious awareness," suggests that operating room conversations might well influence the outcome of surgery.

Hawkeye Pierce, the wry surgeon of M*A*S*H, and some of his real life counterparts in the medical profession should be disturbed by Bennett's findings. They indicate that inadvertent negative remarks and insensitive banter may have an adverse effect on a patient's recovery, whether or not these remarks can be recalled consciously. Such comments as "It's hopeless," "This leg won't work right," or "It may be cancerous," could spell disaster for some patients. Patients seem especially vulnerable to upsetting remarks, as their normal coping mechanisms do not function in their anesthetized state.

At the same time this type of research hints at the promise that deliberate, positive verbal suggestions could have during surgery. Many post-operative complications, such as problems urinating or breathing, have been successfully treated by telling anesthetized patients to breathe deeply afterwards or relax their pelvic muscles after surgery.

"What we are talking about," says Bennett, "is the care of the nervous system during surgery and anesthesia. This care involves providing the nervous system with the food that it thrives on, that is, information. If you don't provide it with information, or provide it with negative information it could be very distressing. Being under anesthesia is sort of like being at a dinner conversation but you can't see, speak or gesture. People talk in rather graphic clinical terms about matters of utmost concern to your survival, but there is nothing you can do or say."

Bennett's studies were inspired by the work of Dr. David Bradley Cheek, a controversial San Francisco gynecologist and hypnotist, who reported that people under hypnosis could recall events from surgery which would help them recover from their traumatic neurosis. "The problem with Cheek's studies," says Bennett, "was that he didn't use the experimental method; it was all anecdotal. He never documented whether the patients' recollections had actually ever taken place. But I think he was right in what he said."

Twenty-five years ago Cheek was saying that "The anesthetized patient may lose all motor reflexes, lose all ability to communicate with the outside world, lose all sense of pain, but. . . [be] able to hear and remember important events at a deep level of subconscious thought." Cheek even went so far as to suggest that every operating room, recovery room and intensive care unit bear a sign that read: "Be Careful, The Patient Is Listening."

Despite the evidence, the medical community remains skeptical and the use of constructive suggestions under anesthesia has yet to acquire the legitimacy of the scalpel and the sponge in the operating room. "People who go into surgery and anesthesia are very concrete sorts of thinkers who think that words are soft and not real medicine," says Bennett. "They also tend to confuse perception and memory. They think that if the patient can't reflect upon, or talk about, his experience under anesthesia, then he is not having any experience. 'As long as the patient can't tell me about it,' they think, 'what difference does it make what I said?'"

Though this attitude may be the rule among physicians, there are exceptions. One is Dr. Bernard Siegel, a surgeon in New Haven, Connecticut with twenty years of experience. For the past five years Siegel has deliberately spoken messages of support to patients under anesthesia.

"People are afraid of anesthesia," says Siegel, "so before the operation I tell my patient's don't worry, we will have contact.

Then during surgery I talk to their unconscious. I tell them what we are finding, I tell them positive things about their problem, I ask them not to bleed, and I tell them they will wake up comfortable, hungry and thirsty. I've found that the attitude of these people is vastly different in the recovery room than those who hear: 'What a mess. This is a catastrophe. If they ever leave here it will be feet first.' Then you wonder why people wake up crying in the recovery room."

Siegel is one of only a handful of physicians who use the unconscious in the healing process. "Most physicians are not trained about what the mind can do and are not aware of its ability to communicate with the body," says Siegel. "They act like mechanics and treat people like cars. You don't ask the car to participate. You change its battery. But if a car had consciousness, you would ask it to help you."

On the horizon, however, are small pockets of encouragement. Frank Guerra, an anesthesiologist and psychiatrist at Denver Presbyterian Hospital, has just launched a newsletter called *Human Aspects of Anesthesia,* which is sent to all anesthesiologists. "My entire thrust is to jar anesthesiologists into the realization that what they are doing has critical psychological significance for their patients," says Guerra. "I would urge anesthesiologists that whether or not they believe that the patient is going to have any kind of perception or memory, to behave as if this were the case."

CLEANLINESS MANIA

Does she seem to be cleaning the house every time you visit? Does he spend hours in the bathroom whenever he goes in for a shower? Does an empty can of deodorant set off the equivalent of a Greek tragedy in the house?

When it comes to cleanliness, the boundary that separates the fastidious from the pathological is rather vague. Cleanliness is a matter of degree, but many Americans seem so obsessed with it that their behavior approaches mania. Howard Hughes' legendary fear of germs is just one example. There are many others, equally strange. Like the man who brushed his teeth with scouring powder to get them extra clean. Or the woman, seen by one psychiatrist, who insisted on spraying her husband's erection with disinfectant before having intercourse.

By all indications, we are a nation of soap-crazed cleanliness freaks. Like automatons, we seem to spend our days, and some nights, cleaning this and cleaning that, ourselves and the domestic spaces around us. Each year we spend more than five billion dollars on cleaning and bathroom items. Yet most of the cleaning and grooming practiced today is essentially ritualistic, meant for display and sexual attraction rather than hygiene. Much of our handwashing, for instance, is done to protect our clothing and the things we handle rather than to clean dirt from our hands. Perhaps the American motto should be revised to read: "In God we dust. And scrub. And wash. And mop. And brush. And sweep."

Every culture in the world has its own notion of what it means to be clean. To Americans, cleanliness is neither a purification of the soul nor environmental neatness, but a personal state defined by lack of body odor, sparkling white teeth, and no ring around the collar. This notion is largely derived from the advertisements of the cleaning products industry. Their promotions give us a standard by which we can judge whether our performance is good enough to feel clean about.

Much of our current concern with personal cleanliness, says Edward T. Hall, the world-renowned anthropologist, can be traced to the so-called sexual revolution, which has made us more aware of our bodies. But the ethnic diversity of our cities, he believes, has played an even larger role in this obsession.

"More than anything else," Hall says, "personal cleanliness is an urban phenomenon. Different diets and habits produce different odors, and when you put them together in a city, people become more aware of one another. It probably was city people who developed the notion that it wasn't right to smell; so in order not to offend anyone, Americans have adopted a common standard of cleanliness—the elimination of the body's olfactory envelope, which still surrounds many equally civilized Europeans. Upward mobility had a lot to do with this." Our mothers always reminded us: "If you smell bad, you won't be successful."

Another factor that had a great impact on the cleanliness craze in America is the availability of plumbing. "When I was young," Hall recalls of the 1930s, "Americans bathed once a week, on Saturday nights." Now less than four U.S. households in every hundred lacks a bath or shower. As a result, Americans now bathe once a day on the average, though as many as ten million of us take more than one bath or shower per day.

Cleanliness becomes pathological when the activity begins to impair other daily functions. Office workers who spend ten minutes of every half hour washing their hands and housewives who fear contamination from doorknobs and TV dials have what psychiatrists call obsessive-compulsive disorders. Fortunately, less than one percent of the population suffers from this anxiety disorder. Its most legendary victim was Howard Hughes. While in Las Vegas, he lived in a room separated from the rest of his apartment by a glass partition to ward off germs.

The compulsion to perform a cleaning ritual, while it may be irrational, is not psychotic, insists Dr. Chet Scrignar, a clinical professor of psychiatry at the Tulane University School of Medicine, in New Orleans, and the author of *Stress Strategies: The Treatment of Anxiety Disorders*. What happens, he explains, is that as people begin thinking of contamination, their anxiety level increases. This is the obsession, the series of repetitive thoughts that generate anxiety. When the anxiety reaches a critical point, the victims feel compelled to begin their ritual, such as hand washing. "They'll tell you it's out of their control, but it's not," he says. "It just seems to be."

Once they give in to the compulsion, however, their anxiety fades quickly, and therein lies the problem. Before long, any anxiety, whether associated with the contaminant or not, can trigger the cleaning ritual.

Psychoanalysis has had little success in treating this disorder, but a form of behavior therapy known as flooding, which Scrignar performs on patients who have been hypnotized, has shown considerable promise. "Flooding means that you don't allow people to engage in the compulsion," he explains. "People complain like crazy but their anxiety goes down. It's not as quick as it would be if they washed, but it works." If the anxiety provoking situation re-created under hypnosis fails, the psychiatrist may take more drastic action—hospitalizing the patient, allowing him to wash his hands in the morning, and then removing the faucet knobs from the sink.

A brief look at the history of cleanliness provides a much needed perspective on our current mania. The ancient Greeks used baths more for health reasons than for the removal of dirt, and in Rome bathing was a social duty to be performed in the company of others. But neither the Greeks nor the Romans used soap. They took hot baths and scraped their bodies with twigs.

One of mankind's oldest known forms of soap was urine, reports Alexander Kira in his classic book, *The Bathroom*. It seems that oxidized urine produces ammonia compounds that are a standard agent for dissolving fats. The first "real" soap, however, was invented by the barbarian Gauls. Made of goat's tallow and beech ashes, it was used as a pomade for the hair, not for washing. By the Middle Ages, people who had not bathed in years might hold conversations through handkerchiefs soaked in perfumes or aromatic herbs. In fact, bathing as a matter of routine private cleanliness did not become fashionable until the mid-1800s. Even at the turn of the century, however, some women still urinated on their hands to clean and soften them.

Bathing is now the cornerstone of the American notion of cleanliness, but its psychology is no simple matter. Or so Dr. Ernest Dichter, founder of the Institute of Motivational Research, in New York, found out in the late 1970s when he was asked by the Armour-Dial Company to analyze the bathing behavior of the American people.

His study showed that people who depend on the shower to wake them in the morning were almost addicted; without it, they reported, their whole day went wrong. For others, it seemed that "the bathing ritual helped generate the hope that this day will be better than the last." Still others savored the sensuous self-discovery involved in bathing. Noted Dichter: "The lathering of one's body—getting all of it covered and then washing it all off—is a form of body culture which comes close to narcissistic self-love."

Many bathers, it seems, took literally the somewhat righteous Protestant dictum that cleanliness is next to godliness. Most adults in the study associated bathing with such rituals as baptism and absolution, among other soul-cleansing rites. Some even saw in bathing a hint of immortality—perhaps because cleanliness suggests smooth skin, an antidote to the wrinkles of old age. Many psychiatrists are aware, in fact, that personal care and grooming is an important step toward recovery in withdrawn and depressed people.

There are, however, a few drawbacks to our mania for cleanliness. It seems, first of all, to encourage a certain passivity. "There won't be any revolution in America," says a character in Eric Linkater's *Juan in America*. "The people are too clean. They spend all their time changing their shirts and washing themselves. You can't feel fierce and revolutionary in a bathroom."

Less significant, but no less worrisome to nature lovers, is that the perfume present in most soaps, after-shave lotions, and deodorants attract mosquitoes, gnats, and black flies. But while attracing insects, fastidiousness can repel spouses, say some psychologists. It seems that unless mates hold compatible standards of cleanliness, a marriage probably will not be happy or long lasting.

Perhaps the most disturbing side effect of cleanliness is that it masks our body odors, in effect throwing a blanket over our sex pheromones, the body's natural aphrodisiacs. King Louis XIV apparently had an instinctive awareness of this, since it is known that he would never let a woman into his bed if she had taken a bath within the previous month.

In the end, our desire to clear the air, clean the sky, wash the wind, and take stone from stone and wash them, to paraphrase T. S. Eliot, can never completely ward off a simple truth: that cleanliness is next to impossible. "What after all is a halo?" says a character in Christopher Fry's *The Lady's Not for Burning*. "It's only one more thing to keep clean."

SELF-HARM

For days, the twenty-two-year-old woman has felt a sense of intolerable dread. "It overwhelms me," she says. "I don't know what to do, but I feel that I must do something." Then panic strikes. She reaches for a razor and makes three cuts on her wrist. She feels immediate relief, no pain. "I feel good now," she says. "I'll be okay for a week. Then it'll start all over again."

The scars covering her body are testimony to previous episodes of self-mutilation. But the woman is neither psychotic nor suicidal. Though consciously self-destructive during these bizarre and gruesome episodes, she does not wish to die. Between the attacks, she functions quite normally.

Because this kind of behavior is distinct from suicide, two psychiatrists at the Medical College of Georgia, in Augusta, have proposed that such cases be regarded as a distinct new category of mental disorder. Doctors E. Mansell Pattison and Joel Kahan call it the Deliberate Self-Harm syndrome, or DSH.

"This is a syndrome of late adolescence," explains Pattison, head of the school's psychiatry department, "in which young people do some type of low-lethality damage to their bodies without the intent to kill themselves. The behavior is then repeated an average of ten-to-fifteen times over a period of eight-to-ten years."

Deliberate self-harm is a world apart from both psychotic and suicidal behavior. To begin with, those who practice DSH behavior do things that, while horrifying, are not life-threatening. They deliberately bite or burn themselves, cut or otherwise mutilate their genitals, even slice off an ear or gouge out an eye or the tongue. Much psychotic and suicidal behavior, by contrast, is marked by one or two episodes in which a person may attempt to perform a potentially fatal act such as shooting or hanging or jumping from a great height.

After analyzing fifty-six cases of self-harm, Pattison and Kahan found there were also differences in age and motivation between the suicide-prone and those with DSH. Suicidal individuals usually are middle-aged—forty-five years old or more—and are plagued with feelings of worthlessness and helplessness. Self-mutilators tend to be much younger and act more from despair, anxiety, or anger.

"Self-harm is also much more prevalent than suicidal behavior," according to Pattison. Each year there are at least four times as many incidents of DSH as there are suicide attempts. But he suspects that his estimate may be too low, because many cases of the syndrome are incorrectly included in the suicide statistics.

While the suicide rate is relatively unchanged over the past two decades, according to Pattison and Kahan, the incidence of deliberate self-harm has increased. One reason, they suggest, is that an ever-increasing number of young people are being placed in penal institutions. "We have more institutionalization today than we had thirty years ago," says Pattison. It is his guess that DSH behavior is a by-product of incarceration. "This is an everyday occurrence in prisons. At a juvenile reformatory, you're likely to see it every couple of days. At a youth detention center, every week. We might be artificially provoking such behavior."

Some cases of self-harm may be overlooked altogether. "Often no one will pick up on them," Pattison notes. The injury will be treated with no thought to what caused it. During the DSH victim's first visit to an emergency room, he might be treated by a surgeon. The next time, he might see an internist, and a year later, an ophthalmologist or dermatologist. "Very few of these cases are referred to a psychiatrist," Pattison says. Even when they are noticed, these people may be dismissed as manipulators, malingerers or attention-seekers, because their self-destructive acts are not lethal.

Self-mutilation, sometimes labeled para-suicide, autoaggression or symbolic wounding, is not a new concept for psychiatrists. (Pattison himself prefers the term *self-harm* to *self-mutilation* because it includes consciously harmful acts that produce no external mutilation: pill swallowing, heavy drinking, even staring straight into the sun. He also draws a clear distinction between deliberate self-harm behavior and ritual mutilation such as head molding, ear-piercing, circumcision, and other socially approved forms of mutilation.) Doctors have usually regarded this sort of behavior as a symptom of the borderline personality disorder, a condition found in people who have not formed strong egos. Yet studies by Pattison and other psychiatrists show no clear association between deliberate self-harm and any specific personality disorder.

The one feature that DSH victims do seem to have in common, notes Pattison, is that they never adequately separated from the nurturant maternal objects—their mothers—at a critical time in their lives. It is during the second year of life that most children first start to notice when their mothers are absent. Typically, a child will become anxious and will search frantically for the mother. If he fails, the child will get depressed and may begin beating and biting and clawing himself. This behavior, according to some psychologists, is the child's misguided attempt to duplicate the mother's physical contact. If the mother returns and holds him, the child's anxiety disappears.

Normal children are usually able to resolve that separation anxiety by the age of three. Those who do not may reexperience this agonizing conflict of individualization and separation from their mothers during late adolescence. This is a particularly vulnerable stage of life, a time when the young person is trying to achieve adulthood and separation from his parents. Conflicts from an earlier age are evoked at this time and the pattern of self-harm may be the result.

Cutting and burning oneself may seem to be farfetched substitutes for maternal contact, but from the DSH victim's point of view, he is experiencing a psychic release. "He focuses on the simulating effects of the contact rather than on the act of inflicting pain," Pattison explains. "Afterwards, he may feel embarrassed or ashamed, but he doesn't feel guilty. 'I can't help it,' he says. 'I have to do this in order to survive.' So we think the act may be an attempt, paradoxically, at self-preservation."

Pattison and Kahan found that certain social factors, such as feeling isolated or having a disruptive family life, seem to provoke deliberate self-harm. Other factors associated with suicidal behavior—the recent loss of someone close or having a serious disease—are not related to DSH, although the syndrome may mark a person as a potential suicide risk.

No one yet understands why it usually takes about a decade for the syndrome to play itself out. But like other kinds of impulsive behavior, self-harm seems to have a kind of burnout phenomenon. "It's as if they have finally begun to learn the lessons of life," Pattison says.

Many psychiatrists seem to feel that Pattison and Kahan have accurately described what is happening to many of their patients. These doctors are in favor of having DSH recognized by the American Psychiatric Association. "About half the cases of self-mutilation that I see fit into this syndrome," says Dr. Armando Favazza, a University of Missouri professor of psychiatry whose book, *Slices of Life,* discusses the broader topic of self-mutilation as a social and psychiatric phenomenon. "I think Pattison is right in saying that we should define DSH as a separate syndrome. That would focus our attention on the behavior so that we might begin to think about what causes it and how to treat it."

For now, the medical establishment is experimenting with different ways to treat this bizarre problem. "We try things," states Favazza in a matter-of-fact tone. "If a patient tends to be a little psychotic, we give him medication. If he tends to be a little depressed, we give him medication. If he is a little anxious, we give him medication. We try and talk with him."

Therapy sometimes helps a person recognize his separation anxiety and learn how to cope with the panic he feels. "Unfortunately," concludes Pattison, "there are no nifty-dandy answers."

HUMAN BITES

An angry Detroit crowd of forty people attacked and bit two emergency-service technicians a few years ago because it took them so long to get to the scene of a traffic accident. Earlier a traveling salesman was found guilty of biting off a woman's nose during an attack in a hotel parking lot in Norfolk, Virginia. And most recently, actor James Garner tried to bite the motorist who grabbed, beat and choked him after a minor traffic accident in Los Angeles.

The growing number of people sinking their teeth into one another is alarming public-health officials who feel that human bites are a serious medical problem. "Human bites are more severe than animal bites," says Dr. Margaret Grossi, deputy commissioner for health in New York City, "because the human mouth has a wider variety of pathogenic organisms." Bites frequently lead to serious complications, the most common being infection, but there is also potential for gross disfigurement, amputation—even death in some cases.

Medical literature has recorded a smattering of such accounts since the beginning of the century, but recognition of human bites as a widespread phenomenon came not long ago, when Dr. John Marr, then epidemiologist and assistant commissioner for preventable diseases in the New York City Department of Health, somewhat whimsically decided to include a category for humans on the city's animal-bite-report form. When the year-end totals for 1977 were tabulated, Marr was shocked to find that 879 incidents of human bites had been reported; each, by definition, had broken skin and drawn blood.

Since then the number of human bites reported in New York City has nearly doubled. The figure jumped to four digits in 1980, with 1,207 bites reported that year. In 1983, the latest year for which figures are available, the number of people who sank their teeth into one another rose to 1,581. Humans now outbite the city's cats, rats, skunks, and parrots. Dogs, of course, bit more people than all those animals put together, but in the same seven-year period the incident of reported dog bites has dropped by almost half.

Humans now account for more than four bites a day in New York, and many bites probably are not being reported. "It is estimated that for every reported dog bite there is also an unreported one," says Martin Kurtz, director of New York City's Bureau of Animal Affairs. "I don't see why we shouldn't expect the same thing with human bites."

Many health officials believe that the increase in biting incidents is a clear indication of the mounting violence in American society. Although New York City is the only place in the United States where human bites are a reportable medical condition, one has every reason to believe that the problem exists nationwide. "I'm sure you would find it to the same degree in cities like Philadelphia, Chicago, and Houston, where there is a lot of crime," says Grossi. "I see no reason why New Yorkers would corner the market on people's biting one another."

Attempts to understand the problem have focused on such questions as when people bite, which parts of the body are usually bitten, and who gets bitten. Like dog bites, human bites show a seasonal pattern, with the largest number occurring in the summer and peaking in July. The hands, fingers, arms, and shoulders are the most likely targets, followed by the face and the neck, with the lower extremities being the least likely targets. Studies also show that males are bitten slightly more often than females. Most victims are fifteen to twenty years old, which is in sharp contrast to dog bites, in which the victims are often less than ten years old.

And just why do people bite people? Marr found that about three-quarters of the New York bite reports were associated with aggressive activities. (Accidents during sports and games accounted for the remainder.) "Usually in fist fighting, or in fighting for one's life, everything comes into play," Marr says.

In self-defense it's pure instinct to use everything as a
weapon—including one's teeth.

The teeth are a formidable weapon in the arsenal of survival,
an effective additional tool to our fists and feet. And no wonder:
The tooth is the human body's sharpest instrument, and tooth
enamel is one of the hardest substances known. A U.S. Special
Forces hand-to-hand expert at Fort Bragg, North Carolina, asserts that biting is not a part of the training, but he would recommend it highly in hand-to-hand combat. Some rape counselors and self-defense instructors say that biting is an effective
tactic against an assailant.

Different groups of people may have different reasons for biting, says Dr. Allan Beck, a former colleague of Marr's in the
Health Department and currently the director of the Center for
Interaction of Animals and Society, in Philadelphia. "Young
adult males are usually the aggressive biters," he says. "Those
are the most aggressive years for everything. They get killed
the most in cars. They get killed the most in homicides."

"Then we have a group of younger people who bite, probably
more in play," Beck continues. "Much of play in primates is pre-
liminary exercise for adult activities, including aggression, and
that's why children play with guns and Barbie dolls. Adult humans bite, too, if someone is punching them or trying to grab
their throat. Cops in scuffles receive a lot of knuckle bites.
Mental-health workers and dentists get bitten, too, for obvious
reasons."

Psychoanalysts consider biting behavior as a regression to
the oral stage of child development. For children the mouth is
also an outlet for aggressive feelings. By the time children
reach the age of two, however, they have usually learned that
biting is not civilized; so they choose to kick and punch instead.
"We all retain characteristics of the oral stage," says the noted
psychiatrist Emmanuel Tanay. "So all of us bite. Some people
bite their nails, some bite into pencils. Sexually stimulating
bites are considered normal, as are those made in self-defense.
It becomes aberrant behavior, however, by the quantity of the
biting and by the nature of the object bitten."

Health officials hope that, by drawing attention to the problem, people will come to understand the seriousness of human
bites. Marr suggests that a systematic examination of the re-

ports of human bites might even serve as a useful index of aggressive and pathological human behavior. "For example," Marr says, "it might point out where a lot of the fistfights are occurring so that the city could allocate more policemen to patrol those areas."

To forensic scientists, bite marks can sometimes be as valuable as a fingerprint. Because no two person's teeth appear to be exactly alike, a suspect's dental pattern can be damning evidence. Several years ago bite-mark evidence led to the conviction of Theodore Bundy, who was accused of bludgeoning and strangling two women at Forida State University. A faint bite mark had been found on the buttocks of one of the women.

Bite marks are common not only in sexual homicides but in child-abuse homicides as well. "Nearly one-fifth of all the children who come to autopsy in New York City have been cannibalized or bitten prior to death," says psychiatrist Judianne Densen-Gerber, J.D., president of the Odyssey Institute, an international public-health-advocacy organization. "We wonder about the children who survive such attacks, those who have had experience after experience of a parent losing control. I have seen enraged parents growl and grit their teeth. Some people really do act like dogs."

From a strictly evolutionary point of view, man's teeth may well be regarded as his oldest weapon. Through the ages combatants drew farther and farther apart as knives gave way to swords, as swords grew longer, and as guns became more accurate. Biting became less common. The caveman and cavewoman probably did more biting than we do. "I have no doubt they did," Beck says. "Apes and monkeys are evidence of that. In fact, I'm sure that if we were to give our monkey friends handguns, they would bite less, too."

TECHNO-JINX

"Oh, no. I can't do that," stammers a woman who has been asked to take some photographs with an instant camera. "Cameras and I just don't get along—it won't work," she explains. Overriding these objections, her employer proffers an Instamatic and shows her how to use it.

In no time at all, however, the woman has broken three cameras. Each camera had produced a good picture when it was demonstrated to her, but each time she tried to take a picture on her own, it had failed. All three cameras ended up at the repair shop. All she could say was: "Can I go now?"

The age of technology is not welcomed by all. Many people repeatedly encounter some quite serious and inexplicable difficulties in their interactions with machines and electronic equipment. Computers crash in their presence, copying machines jam up, watches stop functioning, and telephones won't work.

"Relatively few of these anecdotes have found their way into the literature," notes Robert Morris, an experimental psychologist at Syracuse University who has been studying human performance anomalies of this kind for about three years. "We seem to be dealing with a very informal kind of industrial folklore."

Morris, who resembles a slight, mild-mannered Jack Nicholson with thick glasses, occupies a small office in a rather shabby ten-room suite known as the Communication Studies Laboratory. It is here that he hopes to unravel the puzzle of why people come to regard themselves, or are regarded by others, as linked with the failure of the machinery around them. He refers to such people as malfunction-linked people, or MLPs, for short.

"I call them MLPs," Morris explains, "because I don't want to insult people by calling them jinxes, or hoodoos, or Jonahs, or klutzes. And I want to emphasize that these people are linked to malfunctions; they are not malfunctioning people."

An informal survey, which Morris conducted with a questionnaire he has designed, found that at least one person in ten believes himself or herself to be malfunction-linked. But since the results came from a small sample of people interested in technology Morris expects the proportion of MLPs in the general population may be much greater.

If he is correct, we may soon be faced with a significant social problem, especially as our lives become increasingly involved—if not dependent—on technology. Indeed, there are indications that technostress, as personnel managers sometimes refer to the situation, may already be a problem of considerable magnitude. In Silicon Valley, some psychologists are beginning to specialize in treating people for computerphobia, as well as other kinds of technophobia.

Exactly why technology repeatedly fails for certain individuals is something of a mystery. To find the answer, Morris has begun collecting relevant anecdotes on the subject. Some of the stories involve people who are unable to wear wristwatches, including one individual who went through nineteen new watches before giving up on the idea. Other stories concern such things as computer systems that have a reputation for breaking down just when those most skilled at repairing them are unavailable.

He also found a story in which a person's knack for having things go wrong had reached legendary proportions. Wolfgang Pauli, the Nobel-prize winning theoretical physicist, was apparently so accident-prone that malfunctions occurring in his vicinity were attributed to something called the "Pauli Effect." Writing in the July 1959 *Scientific American,* physicist George Gamow noted that "apparatus would fall, break, shatter or burn when he [Pauli] merely walked into a laboratory."

Of course, accident-proneness has been a familiar concept in the psychological literature since the early part of the century.

Reliability engineers and industrial psychologists have tried to explain all such phenomena in terms of "human factors." They believe that most accidents are simply a matter of a risky job or poor working conditions. Others are due to fatigue, carelessness, and incompetence. Even impulsiveness, aggression and sabotage are thought to play a part. Yet despite such attempts to explain the phenomena, much uncertainty still remains.

Two recent British studies that managed to establish controls for these factors in natural settings could not resolve that uncertainty. In one, at a car manufacturing plant, occupational psychologist A. J. Boyle of the Barking College of Technology found "individuals are differentiated with respect to their accident rates even when there are controls for such factors as ambient risk levels, period of exposure to risk and age and job experience." So it would appear that accident proneness involves still other variables that have so far eluded scientific detection.

That's why Morris is open to the possibility that psychokinesis, or PK, may be at work. PK is the alleged ability of human consciousness to have a specific, concrete effect on the behavior of physical systems.

Morris hit upon this idea quite accidentally while he was running a PK experiment three years ago. The goal of the study was to see whether subjects could influence the behavior of a computerized random-number generator. Because it is widely believed that striving for desired results works against PK, subjects were instructed to adopt an attitude of passive cooperation in their interaction with the equipment. By the time Morris tested thirty-three of sixty-four subjects, however, the computer had crashed in the presence of thirteen people; the experiment was aborted.

At first Morris and his associates joked about whether these subjects had taken their task too seriously. But before examining the attitude questionnaires that the subjects had completed at the start of the experiment, Morris decided to formulate a couple of hypotheses about what might have happened. Perhaps, he thought, the computer had failed in the presence of those subjects who held the more negative attitudes toward psychic phenomena and who were more inclined toward having performance anxiety.

"That's exactly what we found," says Morris. "The thirteen people for whom the computer had crashed were significantly more negative in their attitudes toward psychic abilities. They were also significantly more prone toward anxiety when called upon to perform. Of course, our numbers are very small; so either this is just a statistical aberration of some sort and there really is nothing here, or else we have blundered into something quite important."

Morris later isolated the computer problem to a faulty interface board. The board apparently had several structural flaws, which caused it to malfunction periodically. It is tempting to attribute sole responsibility for the computer crashes to this faulty interface. "But why then," Morris asks, "did it occur so consistently related to the attitudes of the people involved?"

Morris is clearly excited by the prospect of finding a new factor contributing to human-equipment interactions. "But," he states cautiously, "we are fully prepared for the possibility that the anecdotes we have uncovered fall well within the range of presently understood factors."

For now, Morris hopes to begin a project that will enable him to isolate the PK effect in human-equipment interactions, if it actually exists. "The project would allow us to integrate our parapsychological questions into the area of human factors research," he explains. "We want to understand what the range of problems are and tease out the situations which seem to be consistently identified with high rates of equipment malfunction. And if there is a PK effect, we hope to find it by erecting a circumstance in which we understand why the machine is malfunctioning and know that it could not be due to the ordinary means of the person interacting with it."

All psychic phenomena, Morris believes, can be viewed as anomalies of human communication. "Everything that people label as psychic functioning seems to be a matter of information or human influence getting from one place to another in ways that we don't understand," he says.

MLPs are not Morris's only concern, however. He is also trying to understand why certain people tend to be consistently successful in interacting with technology. He calls these people, function-linked people, or FLPs. Who hasn't heard stories about machines that work only when the repairman is present? Unfortunately, such episodes are less likely to be noticed than those associated with malfunction.

Our goal," says Morris, "is to examine how MLPs and FLPs

differ from one another, in order to suggest hypotheses about ways to make the former more like the latter. We hope to be able to intervene and train people to be much more effective when interacting with equipment. We want to help people get along better with the technology that is surrounding them."

While Morris does not see himself as a malfunction-prone person, he does admit to a preference for the non-technical version of things. "When I was four or five years old," he recalls, "I was shocked very badly a couple of times by touching a radio in the kitchen with a wet hand. So I built up this notion that large gray metal boxes with knobs on them could hurt you and the best thing to do was avoid them."

Malfunctions are now Morris's stock-in-trade, but they seldom bring him satisfaction. Like all researchers, he complains of inadequate funding. His work, however, has a particular drawback. "As you can imagine," he says, "having equipment break down all the time tends to get quite expensive."

OF TWO MINDS

Imagine a child playing with blocks. The child decides to build a tower that he can topple. Let's call the destructive agent within the child WRECKER. This agent gets his kicks from knocking over towers and hearing blocks tumble to the floor. To accomplish this goal, WRECKER needs another agent, BUILDER, who will construct a tower.

BUILDER calls on his crew, which includes PUT, who knows how to move a block to a specific location, as well as GRASP, and TRAJECTORY to do the actual construction work. The blocks begin to stack up. But eventually a conflict arises between BUILDER, who wants to make the tower even higher, and WRECKER, who is satisfied with its height and wants to knock it over. There to arbitrate the conflict is their superior agent, PLAY-WITH-BLOCKS, a minion of yet another agent named PLAY, whose idea this was in the first place.

But PLAY himself quickly becomes engaged in a conflict with I'M GETTING HUNGRY. Once this agent gets control, the structure that PLAY has organized starts to disintegrate. Yet before fading out completely, WRECKER manages to eke out a victory by smashing the tower on the child's way out to the kitchen.

The original version of this remarkable scenario, designed to illuminate what may be occurring beneath the surface of the child's mind, was created by Marvin Minsky, one of the chief architects of the field of artificial intelligence, in collaboration with Seymour Papert, a professor of education and mathematics at Massachusetts Institute of Technology who spent several years working with child psychologist Jean Piaget. Their scenario illustrates a view of the mind quite at odds with the traditional concept of the self as a single agent.

Minsky and Papert argue that the mind is composed of many smaller minds, which are themselves composed of yet smaller minds. These minds, or agents, and the interconnections between them, form a society known as the self. This theory, which they call The Society of Minds, is one of the new ideas about ourselves and the way we think that have emerged since the field of artificial intelligence began flirting with the jealously guarded topics of psychology just two and a half decades ago.

"There must be several hundred ideas that are new under the sun which psychology never had," says MIT professor Minsky, reflecting on the computer's influence on studies of the mind. His work in psychology, psycholinguistics, and epistemology these days is such that many see him as more of a philosophical psychologist than a computer scientist. "Computers helped us develop ideas about how to describe complicated processes," he continues, "and there never were any precise ones before computers. That's why psychology was stuck. With these new ideas, we can now ask about mental phenomena and think about how they could actually work. That's not to say we now know how they actually do work, but at least for the first time we are able to propose ways in which they might work, and ways in which machines might do such things. That's the great revolution."

The revolution is as much a conceptual change in our understanding of man as it is a technological change to a new world of intelligent machines. The instrument of change is not the plow this time, or the assembly line, but the computer. It has told us more about ourselves than any other psychological tool—the maze, the electric shock, the stopwatch—ever did. For the first time explorers of the mind have been able to test their theories with computer simulations of human cognitive processes. The computer may well be the best instrument to study the mind since the mind itself.

Artificial intelligence is the science of making machines that think. To insiders, this relatively new branch of computer science is known simply as "AI." A good deal of work in AI is based on having machines mimic human intelligence, though the majority of researchers are more concerned about how well a task can be performed regardless of the way humans do it. Progress in the field has been slower than expected, but the cause for the delay does not appear to be one of technology. It seems to have more to do with a lack of understanding about ourselves.

Quite unexpectedly, the attempt to program intelligence into the computer has led researchers back to the study of human intelligence. This effort on the part of AI researchers, along with the work of their colleagues in the allied field of cognitive science, has produced a wealth of new insights about the workings of the human mind.

AI's track record is already quite impressive. For instance, we might have known that our short-term memories could hold very little information, but until we had to deal with the problem of information storage and retrieval in intelligent machines, we never suspected how this apparent limitation helped us deal with the present and anticipate the future. We have always thought of ourselves as good educators, but we never realized how confused we really were about the learning process until we tried to teach machines how to learn on their own. We have always boasted about the supremacy of human expertise, our mathematical ability, our ability to play chess, to diagnose diseases, only to realize how relatively easy it is for machines to mimic these types of human performance. And much to our surprise, we have learned that one of the things keeping us a step ahead of the machines at the moment is that human quality which we so often take for granted, good old common sense. The ways of the mind, we have discovered, are not nearly as mysterious as we once believed.

So many of the computer's activities resemble human cognitive processes that the comparison between man and machine has never been more apt. Never mind that the brain's architecture is different from that of the computer; never mind that wetware (read: brain cells) is not hardware. Both mind and machine accept information, manipulate symbols, store items in memory and retrieve them again. Whether machines do these things like people do is less significant than the fact that they do them at all.

"Obviously people don't think the same way as machines," says Seymour Papert. "People are biological. When we ask if a machine thinks, we are asking whether we would like to extend the notion of thinking to include what machines might do. That is the only meaningful sense of the question: Do machines think? When Newton said the Sun exerts a force on the Earth he introduced a new technical concept of force. Artificial intelligence, in a similar way, is introducing a new technical concept of thinking."

The era of the human being as the measure of all things has ended. Already AI scientists suspect that intelligent behavior is shaped as much by the problem itself as by the problem solver's own abilities. The outcome of such thinking will not be a theory of human intelligence or a theory of machine intelligence, but a general theory of intelligence, regardless of whether it is realized in silicon or tissue. This lumping together of man and machine inevitably creates some uneasiness. But, as Papert points out, just as a real understanding of bird flight came from an understanding of flight, not birds, a real understanding of human intelligence is more likely to come from an understanding of intelligence, not human beings.

"We are to thinking as the Victorians were to sex," Papert told Pamela McCorduck, the author of *Machines Who Think,* a fascinating history of artificial intelligence. Everyone does it, but no one knows how to talk about it. The study of artificial intelligence has introduced more structure into our thinking about thinking. The vocabulary of the field has enabled scientists to be more specific about the different ways in which the mind might work. This new langugage of thought is proving to be particularly well-suited for constructing psychological theories.

"Prior to the computer age," says Princeton University professor George Miller, a noted cognitive psychologist, "psychologists sort of had a choice between being vague and being wrong. You could be psychoanalytic and talk vaguely about the id and the ego and the superego. Or you could talk about conditioned reflexes, which may hold for rats and fishes but are not very good models for men, and you could be quite precise and undoubtedly wrong. Then the computers came along and they gave us a language in which we could formulate more interesting theories. Even better, we could run these theories on the computer and we could have a chance to see what would happen and what the theory's implications were. This was an enormous step forward in freeing the imaginations of psychologists."

Early in the history of artificial intelligence researchers were firmly convinced that a few underlying principles characterized all kinds of intelligent human behavior, and that once these principles were elucidated they could then be utilized in making intelligent machines. Their belief in the universality of these principles meant that the laws of thought could be isolated from any problem-solving task, whether it was playing a game of chess, finding the shortest route to the grocery store, or solving a mathematical puzzle.

The principles they uncovered helped to clarify a handful of age-old procedures which humans use for solving problems. These include "generating and testing" (Does this work? If not, try something else) and "means-ends analysis" (Look at the present situation and the goal; then try to reduce the differences between the two). These and other principles eventually made their way into many of the creativity and problem-solving seminars that abound in schools and businesses today.

Before long, however, many researchers became convinced that these universal principles were not sufficient to produce programs that accurately mimicked intelligent human behavior. What the programs lacked, they discovered, was knowledge. Not general knowledge, but specialized knowledge, and lots of it. Specialized knowledge is that messy bunch of details and rules of thumb drawn from experience and good judgment. This realization gave rise to a new hybrid, a machine that integrated some general strategies of problem solving with a large base of knowledge specific to the problem at hand. A few models of this new breed of intelligent machines, known as expert systems, are beginning to take their place in human affairs.

Expert systems attempt to simulate human performance within a limited area of knowledge. This specialization means that a program designed to select antibacterial agents for treating infections cannot deal with a broken leg, and that as far as a chess program is concerned a game of checkers looks no different than a Martian princess.

Some expert systems can read and summarize news stories, write poetry, compose music, counsel investors, give psychiatric tests, or direct the flow of parts and materials in a factory. Others are far better than any human at routing air traffic, analyzing cardiograms, selecting the most likely sites for oil wells, performing symbolic integration in calculus, and elucidating chemical hypotheses. One of the most impressive of all expert systems is a program named CADUCEUS, which can diagnose hundreds of diseases in internal medicine as well as most practiced physicians.

These systems are labelled "expert" because their behavior suggests that they are knowledgeable about a particular domain. Each such system contains two types of knowledge. The first is factual knowledge, which is commonly agreed upon and is easy to program for computer use. *Ripe bananas are yellow.* The other type is heuristic knowledge. This is the knowledge of experience and good judgment. Heuristics are the rules of thumb of a particular field. *When making a right turn on a bicycle, lean left.* This type of knowledge is largely private and lies buried within the minds of those with the know-how. It must be mined by people known as knowledge engineers.

These engineers manage to extract heuristic knowledge from experts by having them talk aloud about how they go about solving the problems in their particular speciality. The knowledge engineers can then translate the procedures that experts use to solve problems into the formal language of computer programming. (These programs are often written in the form of if-then rules: *If the whites of the patient's eyes are yellow, then he has a buildup of bile pigments in his body.*) This sort of mining operation can take several months or several years. The endproduct is an expert system. The by-product is a glimpse into the nature of human knowledge and human thinking.

"One of the things we've learned in developing expert systems is that we do not necessarily go about solving problems the way we think we do," says Randall Davis of the Artificial Intelligence Laboratory at MIT. He recalls the surprise that a doctor expressed when his explanation of a diagnostic solution failed to work on the machine. "What he had told us, in other words, turned out not to be the way he must really be doing it. We have many experiences like that. The need to be very precise has forced us to examine much more carefully what in fact we think we do. There's the old joke about not really understanding something until you have taught it to somebody else. The new version now says that you don't really understand it until you've programmed it into a computer."

The new intelligent machines have also managed to strip expertise of much of its sacred aura. "Many of the things that seemed mysterious to us before, like intuition, aren't quite so mysterious when you really sit down to examine them," says Davis. "Many people would say that Jack Myers and Harry Pople's new program in internal medicine (formally known as CADUCEUS, and jokingly referred to as JACK-IN-THE-BOX) has captured some of the intuition of a good intelligent medical diagnostician. In fact, whether or not they have captured the intuition is less important for an expert system than the fact that they have captured some of the performance."

It seems that human experts seldom engage in formal deductive reasoning, and rarely does anyone else, for that matter. Even though we have considered ourselves champions in this respect ever since Aristotle, it turns out that computers are far superior to humans when it comes to this kind of abstract reasoning.

"We think that humans reason more by example," says cognitive psychologist Donald Norman, who is director of the Institute for Cognitive Science at the University of California at San Diego. "We rarely think or make decisions by standard rules of logic. Human reasoning seems to operate more by means of analogy and experience. The physician prescribing a drug seems to forgo logical analysis until he has reached his solution by other means. He will first try to recall the last few patients with symptoms resembling those of his present patient and then try to remember whether or not the drugs prescribed for those patients were beneficial to them."

Experts only seem to use deductive logic when explaining their solutions to others or to confirm those solutions for themselves. The novice, on the other hand, seems to resort to it regularly, probably out of desperation for a way to generate answers.

Novices and experts differ in other unexpected ways as well. "What separates one from the other, isn't what you might think," says John Anderson, a professor of psychology and computer science at Carnegie-Mellon University in Pittsburgh, one of the three major centers for AI research in the United States, with MIT in Cambridge and Stanford University in California. Anderson is viewed by many as a leading theoretician of thinking. "In chess, for instance, there isn't much difference between the duffer and the master in overall intelligence, and both will consider the same number of moves. What distinguishes the master is that he has committed to memory the appropriate analysis of the tens of thousands of patterns that possibly could occur on the chessboard."

These patterns, or combinations of information, allow the master to quickly recognize situations and deal with them according to experience. "It seems that a major component of being intelligent," Anderson says, "is based on this ability to convert as much of one's knowledge into knowledge that can be used in pattern matching. This is what we think happens when someone becomes an expert in a field."

This conversion of knowledge may be directly responsible for much of the expert's efficiency in applying knowledge, as well as his difficulties in making it explicit. Learning a foreign language is a dramatic example of this process. In the classroom we are first taught the rules of the language. But our ability to speak is very slow at first because we are constantly having to call these rules to mind and figure out how they apply to the current situation. Once we become fluent, however, we no longer have to recall the rules, and it is often the case that we forget what the rules are. The more we lose conscious access to our knowledge, the better we seem to become at applying it.

Applying knowledge, however, is not the same as acquiring it. "Expert systems really are wonderful," says Minsky. "I think it surprised everybody what such a small amount of knowledge could do. But expert systems are also very strange and primitive because they don't get better at things, and they don't do anything else. So the question is do they represent half the human mind or just five percent? Nobody knows. But smart people sense that just collecting knowledge isn't the whole thing. Learning is the important thing in the long run. Why can't we have these machines learn on their own?"

The learning problem is one of the major concerns in artificial intelligence. To answer Minsky's question, researchers have gone back and studied how humans learn. Models of children learning geometry problems and language reveal that we do not simply soak up knowledge like sponges.

"What has emerged," Anderson says, "is basically a set of principles of how we learn from doing. It turns out that we learn formal skills like solving problems in physics and doing proofs in geometry not by reading a textbook and understanding the abstract principles, but by actually solving problems in those fields. What the textbooks don't teach you is when to apply the knowledge and that knowing turns out to be about three-quarters of the learning problem."

To learn is to construct a growing network of concepts in the mind, according to a theory of semantic memory developed several years ago by Carnegie-Mellon graduate student M. Ross Quillian. The theory, which views the mind as an enormously complicated and constantly changing network of nodes and links, arose as he tried to construct a computer-search technique based on a model of the human brain.

According to Quillian, when we experience something new, like seeing an exotic animal, we store the information and later retrieve it through a technique called "spreading activation." This means that new material is processed by being linked with previously established ideas or nodes. That way the new animal is not only classified according to form, color, odor and behavior but linked to other animals and a repertoire of feelings and recollections.

This rich network of connections in human memory is one of the most profound differences between humans and machines. The brain's ability to search for information through its millions of neurons simultaneously looks positively uncanny. "Spreading activation makes use of the associations among ideas," Anderson says, "so that when a conversation turns to restaurants, for instance, all the knowledge related to the subject becomes instantly available." Quite unlike the computer, the more information we have about a subject, the faster we seem to be able to retrieve it.

That kind of quick access depends heavily on how the information is stored in the first place. "Careless storage means access will be limited, undependable and slow," explains Dedre Gentner, a cognitive scientist who keeps close tabs on developments in artificial intelligence through her friends at MIT. Gentner studies aspects of learning, comprehension and meaning, and develops mental models of the physical world for Bolt, Beranek & Newman, a research firm in Cambridge, Mass. "When you rig an experiment so that people are forced to store information very quickly and thoughtlessly, they can't get at it again. But if you give people the time to learn, they will organize their knowledge systematically so that retrieval is more reliable."

Yet, as we all know, access to information in human memory is less than ideal at times. Humans are forgetful. Information sometimes gets lost because we break up experiences into bits and pieces and store them in different parts of memory, according to Roger Schank, a professor of computer science and psychology at Yale. But on the positive side, he notes that this breaking up of kowledge in memory also allows us to make better generalizations and more useful predictions.

Human imperfections may be there for a reason. The fact that our short-term working memories are quite small, as psychologists have known for sometime, may be inextricably linked to our high intelligence. "These short memories," Minsky says, "may force us to be smart about things. I think that a number of our limitations are tricks that Nature uses to make us find clever ways of doing things. *If I can't remember where I parked my car, I can usually figure out where I might have parked it because I'm in Technology Square in Cambridge, and on Tuesdays I can usually find a parking space over there.* So even though I may not be able to remember where it is, I can figure it out." A computer with a huge memory would not bother to figure out where the car might be; it would simply look on its disk to find the car's location. Large memories may make for lazy thinkers.

Artificial intelligence has managed to turn many of our precious self-concepts upside down. Look at what it has done to our notions of intelligence. "As soon as the computer is able to do something," Anderson says, "we no longer tend to see that as intelligent. Twenty-five years ago we thought the stuff that it took to do symbolic integration in calculus was real intelligence. Now there are programs that outperform humans at that particular task. So we are now less impressed by the ability to do symbolic integration and probably reasonably so. On the other hand, things that seemed to us initially to be low level and almost trivial in some sense have turned out to be profound in many ways. We are now much more impressed by our ability to hold a conversation and our ability to understand what a scene is just by looking at it."

This apparent paradox has led Minsky to ask in an article called "Why People Think Computers Can't": "Why were we able to make AI programs do such grown-up things before we could make them do childish things?" He thinks perhaps that it is because adult or expert thinking is often somehow simpler than ordinary common sense.

Common sense can be quite tricky. To have a robot deal with children's blocks well enough to stack them up, take them down, rearrange them, and put them in boxes, Stanford University computer scientist Terry Winograd had to develop a new kind of programming, one that was less centralized and more interactive than previous programs. In order to understand the sentence "Pick up the block," one part of the robot program had to figure out if "pick" was a verb, while another part of the program tried to figure out if "block" was the sort of thing that could be picked up. That simple task is enough to illustrate the complexity of common sense reasoning. It seems to require an awful lot of switching back and forth between points of view and different kinds of ideas.

Why has common sense been so hard to achieve in machines? Minsky thinks it's because we are asking the wrong question. Instead of asking what line of thought produced a good decision, we should be asking what prevented us from making a bad decision. He believes that the mind, in order to succeed, must know how to avoid the most likely ways to fail. So he borrows from Freud the concept of censors to explain how the mind avoids making certain blunders. We not only accumulate censors for social taboos and repressions, he says, but also for knowing what is not proper to do in ordinary activities.

"I think that common sense is more a management problem than a knowledge problem," says Minsky. "You need a vast amount of knowledge for common sense, but what is missing in AI theories at the moment is the kind of thing the businessman knows about setting up a large company. There have to be networks of communication, and very little is known about how to make them in artificial intelligence. Among the things that aren't known is how to transmit as little information as possible. The vice-president of manufacturing doesn't want to know how many drill presses there are in Idaho, for instance. So the really important thing in intelligence might be a matter of how often should this agent or department report to the other. If it reports every day, they'll all go crazy. If it reports every six months, the warehouse may go empty before anyone notices."

If the development of common sense in machines appears complex, imagine how difficult it might be to program exotic thinking, such as creativity, into a machine. But Minsky thinks this will actually turn out to be relatively easy to do. He believes that we take ordinary thinking so much for granted that we never wonder how it happens until a particularly unusual performance attracts attention. Then we call it genius or creativity. But there is no substantial difference, he says, between ordinary thought and creative thought. What actually seems to separate the ordinary thinker from the extraordinary thinker is that one has learned to be better at learning. If that is all there is to it, he says, then once we can get machines to learn—and learn to learn better—then one day we might see creativity happening in machines.

Once ordinary human thinking has been programmed into a machine, Minsky believes that even "hard things" like emotions will be programmable. "It is a mistaken idea in our culture that feeling and emotion are deep, whereas intelligence, how we get ideas, how we think, is easy to understand," he says, stroking the crown of hair on his nearly bald head. "If you ask someone, 'Why are you mad at your wife?' they might say, 'Well, it's really because my boss was mean to me, and I can't get mad at him.' It seems to me that people understand the dynamics of emotions quite well. But they have no idea at all to speak of about how thought works. If you asked someone who just got an idea for an eight-wheeled vehicle that would go over bumps easier, 'How did you get that idea?' they are likely to say: 'Well it just popped into my head,' or 'Oh, I just thought of it.' Isn't that shocking? That's the best we can say."

"I think we'll be able to program emotions into a machine once we can do thoughts," he says. "We could make something that just flew into a rage right now, but that would be a brainless rage. It wouldn't be very interesting. I'm sure that once we can get a certain amount of thought, and we've decided which emotions we want in a machine, that it won't be hard to do."

Sherry Turkle, a sociologist at MIT and the author of *The Second Self,* believes that the computer is promoting this type of self-reflection throughout our culture. "It has brought into public debate questions that have been the province of philosophers, psychoanalysts, mystics and theologians," says Turkle, letting her telephone answering machine pick up her calls as she talks. "There's something about working with thinking machines that makes you start thinking about thinking."

Turkle has interviewed hundreds of children and adults in an attempt to gauge the impact of the computer's presence on people, not as a tool for performing calculations, but as an evocative object. "The culture we live in has been called a culture of narcissism," she continues, "but I don't think that captures the anxiety we feel. We are insecure in our understanding of ourselves, and this insecurity has bred a new preoccupation with the question of who we are. The computer is a new mirror, the first psychological machine."

Turkle tells of a group of young children, playing with a computer-controlled tic-tac-toe game at the beach. When a boy named Robert loses to the machine, he accuses it of cheating. A little girl objects: to cheat, she says, you have to know you are cheating, since knowing is part of cheating. They begin discussing whether the machine is alive. They wonder if the machine is conscious, if it can have feelings. Eventually even the youngest children come to realize that the key is emotion rather than motion, psychological rather than mechanical.

"Many adults follow essentially the same paths as these children when they talk about human beings in relation to these new psychological machines," Turkle explains. "They say they are perfectly comfortable with the idea of mind as machine. They even assert that simulated thinking is thinking. But they cannot bring themselves to propose further that simulated feeling is feeling. Somehow they feel compelled to isolate as their core something which is essentially human."

Turkle draws a parallel between the present situation and the post-Darwinian era. "Most people accepted the idea that we are animals," she says, "but they also found a way to think of themselves as something more as well. We learned to see ourselves as rational animals. Now there is the possibility for a new integration, to see ourselves as emotional machines."

Powerful theories of mind always seem to evoke new views of ourselves. The success of another powerful theory of mind, psychoanalysis, had little to do with its validity as a science, says Turkle, whose previous project analyzed the psychoanalytic revolution in France. "The most important factor, I believe, had to do with the power of its psychology of everyday life. Freud's theories of dreams, jokes, puns and slips allowed people to take it up as a fascinating plaything. And the theory was evocative: It gave people a way to think about themselves, and to do it differently than they had done it before. Interpreting dreams and slips allowed people to have contact with taboo preoccupations, to have contact with their sexuality and aggressivity, to have contact with their unconscious wishes."

Turkle's interpretation of the power of the computer's cultural impact rests on its ability to do something of the same sort. "If behind people's fascination with Freudian theory there was a nervous—often guilty—preoccupation with the self as sexual," she says, "behind the increasing interest in computational interpretations of mind is an equally nervous preoccupation with the self as a machine. Our anxiety about the computer is based not so much on whether computers could ever think like people, but on whether people have always thought like computers, and if so, is that the most important and characteristic thing about being human?"

But where psychoanalysis drew our attention to meaning, the computer revolution is drawing our attention to mechanism. "When Freud looked at slips," Turkle says, "he looked at underlying meaning and unconscious motivations. When we look at slips as information-processing errors, we say that we are looking at the same thing, but in fact we are looking at mechanism, how the program got derailed. Some people find this utterly plausible; it sounds reasonable. That's what I mean when I talk about people beginning to accept in some measure that they are machines. But if people really do start thinking of their slips as information-processing errors, that's really a radically different way of looking at our behavior."

Minsky is perhaps the strongest advocate of this new view of human behavior. "I think that what we have learned is that we are probably computers," he says, playfully argumentative. "What that means is that if we don't like how we work, then someday we are gong to be able to intervene. Of course, psychoanalysts said that too, and they were wrong. It wasn't the great breakthrough they thought it would be."

Looking at a complex process such as intelligent behavior and seeing it as the result of many simpler subprocesses is indeed different; it may be oversimplified as well. But there is a new twist to this computer-illustrated reductionism. No longer is it just a matter of taking the clock apart and listing its pieces. We must be able to put the clock, or the person, back together again, and that involves understanding how the pieces fit together as well. The computer has shown the value of connections, that simple things combined can result in something quite sophisticated, but only when put together in the right way. Rather than making the mind less interesting, these attempts to analyze the way we humans think have revealed a complexity that grows more intriguing the more we discover.

LIFE

NEW SOUP OF LIFE

Long ago, when the Earth was young, the land rumbled with active volcanoes, and the sky swarmed with thick, moist clouds that rained until oceans covered much of the globe. It was that special kind of place. Within half a billion years the myriad conditions necessary for the development of life would be met.

Trying to unravel just how life came to exist on this planet has been one of science's most fundamental and perplexing problems. Scientists, working some four billion years after the event, have come to believe that the elemental building blocks of life (amino acids, purines and pyramidines, sugars and fats) arose in the Earth's primordial broth through the action of lightning and sunlight on simple atmospheric molecules. For the past three decades they have assumed that the recipe for this soup of life contained ammonia, methane, hydrogen and water. But recently they have come to a new consensus about the composition of the early atmosphere. The cosmic cookbook is being rewritten.

The man making some of the most substantial contributions to this new view is Dr. Joel Levine, a forty two-year-old atmospheric scientist at NASA's Langley Research Center in Hampton, Virginia. "The overwhelming majority of chemical-evolution experiments since the first one, done thirty years ago, may have been conducted with the wrong atmospheric mixture," he says. "None of the experiments included oxygen, which we believe was present in at least small quantities. And until recently no one was aware of the high levels of ultraviolet radiation that the young sun most probably emitted. These levels are lethal to living systems as we know them.

How could life have formed and evolved in such a hostile environment?"

Levine began his detective work a decade ago, while he was developing a series of sophisticated, computer-based photochemical models designed to assess the impact of man's activities on the composition and chemistry of the atmosphere. (Photochemistry deals with chemical reactions initiated or assisted by exposure to photons, which are elementary particles of light.) Though these models were made to project into the future, Levine became intrigued by the idea of running them backward in time to see what he could learn about the origin and evolution of our atmosphere. That's how NASA got itself into the business of studying the Earth's prebiological atmosphere and how Levine joined the ranks of origin-of-life researchers.

The modern foundations of research into the chemical evolution of life date back to the 1920s, when a Russian biochemist A.I. Oparin and the British geneticist J.B.S. Haldane independently proposed that organic molecules could not have formed in an oxidizing atmosphere (i.e., one containing oxygen molecules). Organic compounds could only form, they believed, in an atmosphere rich in methane, ammonia, hydrogen and water. Their theory of an oxygen-free, or highly-reducing, atmosphere was placed on firm footing in 1952, when a graduate student at the University of Chicago, named Stanley Miller, was prompted by Harold Urey, the late Nobel chemist, to conduct his now-famous experiment. Miller sent a continuous electrical charge through a mixture of methane, ammonia and hydrogen that he circulated through a flask of water vapor. A week later he found that the reddish-brown soup that had formed at the bottom of his collection chamber actually contained several amino acids—the precursors of living systems that had been predicted by Oparin.

Thirty years later, when Levine and his postdoctorate fellow Tommy Augustsson entered the classic mixture of gases into the computer models, they discovered that an early atmosphere with appreciable amounts of methane and ammonia would have been chemically unstable and hence very short-lived. Owing to the decomposing influence of solar ultraviolet radiation and the hydroxyl radical, a molecule that results from the breakup of water vapor, the lifetimes of ammonia and methane would have been less than one hundred years, Levine insists, if they existed at all.

Then what divine breath infused the atmosphere? "That," says Levine, "turns out to have a very simple answer." It has been conveniently provided by the fledgling science of comparative planetology. After a decade and a half of planetary exploration, scientists have come to believe that the atmospheres of Earth, Venus and Mars all formed through the volcanic emission of gases originally trapped during the formation of the planets 4.6 billion years ago. (Temperature differences explain how the three planets could begin with identical compositions yet develop quite different present-day atmospheres.) These volcanic emissions were composed of about 80 percent water vapor, 10 percent carbon dioxide and one percent nitrogen, the remainder being sulfur compounds, chlorine and so on.

So planetary evolution prescribed that the Earth's prebiological atmosphere would be composed primarily of water vapor, carbon dioxide and nitrogen. Recent laboratory lightning experiments by Levine and others suggest that such a mixture can yield life's vital organic compounds. "We have found that all of the gaseous precursors needed for the production of the complex organic molecules, which Urey and Miller formed in their methane, ammonia and hydrogen atmosphere, can also be produced in a carbon dioxide, nitrogen and water-vapor atmosphere," says Levine. "The only difference is that the yields we get are less. But to my way of thinking that just means that it took a little longer, and time is one thing you have when you are talking about hundreds of millions of years."

Another area in the traditional theory of the origin of life that has been thrown into question by Levine and his colleagues is the level of oxygen in the prebiological atmosphere. Until a few years ago, researchers believed that the early atmosphere contained little or no oxygen. The small amounts present were produced through the chemical decomposition of the atmospheric carbon dioxide and water vapor by solar ultraviolet radiation (UV). But it now appears that the early atmosphere may have contained a million times more oxygen than anyone had believed before.

The theoretical insight for this astonishing idea was provided by Vittorio Canuto, an astrophysicist at the Goddard Institute for Space Studies, when he asked Levine how his model of the early atmosphere would be affected by the possibility that the sun had, in its youth, emitted more UV than it does today. According to recent measurements of a half a dozen young sun-like stars, obtained by the observational astronomer Catherine Imhoff using the International Ultraviolet Explorer satellite, the young sun may have emitted as much as ten thousand times more UV than it does today. When Levine inserted the increased UV values into his model, he found that the oxygen levels in the early atmosphere rose by a factor of about one million.

The early geological record appears to support this conclusion. Geologists have long suspected that the oxygen level in the early atmosphere had to be much greater than previously calculated. In their analysis of the oldest known rocks, estimated to be more than 3.5 billion years old, they found oxidized iron and uranium in amounts that called for the atmospheric oxygen levels to be from a hundred to a billion times greater than generally accepted. But according to scientists who study the effects of oxygen as a lethal agent on early life forms, even Levine's calculated millionfold increase in oxygen does not raise the early atmosphere's oxygen level enough to be detrimental to life's emerging organic compounds.

Though some scientists have come to accept the idea of a mildly-reducing atmosphere such as Levine's as the most likely scenario for the origin of life, a heated debate continues regarding the amounts of certain compounds, such as hydrogen, that were present. When asked to comment on Levine's scenario, Stanley Miller, who is now a professor of chemistry at the University of California, San Diego, replied: "If that atmosphere doesn't contain any molecular hydrogen, then no organic compounds will be made." Levine agrees. "There is no question that hydrogen had to be around," he says, "but it was present in very insignificant concentrations compared to the water vapor, nitrogen and carbon dioxide in the early atmosphere."

"All those discussions leave me cold," says John Oro, a professor of biochemistry at the University of Houston and associate editor of the highly respected *Journal of Molecular Evolution.* "There are difficulties in assuming that the Earth produced sufficient amounts of these volatile substances by volcanic outgassing alone." Back in 1961, Oro proposed that comets may have been responsible for depositing these volatiles, and now scientists, including Levine, are beginning to take the suggestion seriously.

While our knowledge of the origin and evolution of the early atmosphere is still incomplete, Levine's colleagues were quick to recognize the value of his accomplishments. The New York Academy of Sciences selected him for the 1982 Halpern Award in Photochemistry, citing his work on the photochemistry of the Earth's atmosphere and its evolution over geological time. He is not only the youngest person to receive the award, but also the first government scientist to be selected.

"I think Levine has made a significant advance," says Oro, one of the world's leading authorities on chemical evolution, though he likes to point out that Darwin, back in 1871, also believed that a mildly-reducing atmosphere was most appropriate for the evolution of the first life forms. "Through a continuation of Levine's work," Oro concludes, "we should one day have a clearer notion of the evolution of the Earth's atmosphere."

PLANTS THAT HEAL

A little headache. A slight burn. A case of constipation. It does not take much for modern man to sing praise to the wonder drugs of western medicine. When things get more serious, rheumatism let's say, or kidney and heart disease, well then thank God, we say, for those tiny pills. Little do we realize, however, just how many of the prescription and over-the-counter drugs we consume every year are actually derived from plants that have been part of the traditional healer's pharmacopoeia for centuries.

"Literally all the wonder drugs on the market from the past forty years or so," says Dr. Edward Ayensu, the distinguished director of Smithsonian's office of biological conservation, "were derived from plant materials and have a long history of use by traditional healers. Take quinine, for instance. Look at the magic it has performed. You know what it is? It's the bark of cinchona, which the Indians chewed when they had malaria. All that we have done is taken it, refined it and made it look nice. But the important thing to realize is that in order to synthesize something you must know its chemistry. And where did we get the knowledge of that chemistry? It didn't come from the heavens. It came from the plant."

Ayensu's interest in medicinal plants dates back almost forty years, when as a young boy living in the western province of Ghana in Africa he witnessed a personal demonstration of the healing power of plants. He had developed a persistent case of acute abdominal pain that showed no response to hospital medication. So his mother took him to a local herbalist who went out into the field to obtain several leaves and the bark of a tree. An attendant then prepared a decoction for him that tasted very bitter, but which, within three days, had stopped his abdominal pains completely.

While Ayensu's experience may seem quite foreign to those of us accustomed to the ways of western medicine, more than three-quarters of the world's people still depend on such herbal medicines and traditional healers for health care, according to the World Health Organization (WHO). The fields of botany and medicine have been synonymous throughout human history. Or so it was until the turn of the twentieth century, when chemists and pharmacologists learned how to synthesize medicinally-active substances and grew contemptuous of folk remedies and drugs of plant origins.

But the field of herbal medicine has seen a renaissance in the past decade, fostered primarily by the enthusiasm and hard work of researchers in the field of natural products. Their members include botanists, such as Ayensu, who search throughout the globe for medicinal lore relating to plants, as well as pharmacognosists and phytochemists, who study plant chemistries and attempt to isolate their active, or medicinal, properties in the laboratory. The aim of these natural product advocates is to discover new active ingredients in nature that might have some potential as a source of drugs.

Of course, not all drugs come from plants. Among the most notable exceptions are the antibiotics, which are derived from microorganisms, and the chemotherapeutic agents, which are sulfur-based. But altogether about half of all the prescription drugs on the market are derived from plants. Perhaps the best example is aspirin. This familiar cure-all is derived from willow bark, which has a long history as a folk remedy to help reduce fevers and aches. During the nineteenth century chemists determined its active ingredients and then synthesized the first aspirin tablets.

Other examples abound. For thousands of years Hindu healers have been using the root of the mandrake plant to treat nervous disorders. But it was not until 1947 that western scientists began to use synthesized extracts of the plant's active ingredient, called reserpine, in the treatment of hypertension and anxiety. Diogenin, a drug used as the starting material in the manufacture of birth control pills, comes from the Mexican yam, a climbing vine long used by Mexican Indians as a general cure-all. And Vincristine, a chemical derived from the Madagascar periwinkle, has led to a remarkable decrease in the mortality rate of young leukemia patients.

Despite such successes scientists still tend to dismiss the effectiveness of herbal medicines because so many traditional healers employ magic and spiritual forces to aid their plant cures. So what Ayensu and others in the field of natural products are trying to do is separate the incantations associated with traditional cures from the chemistry of the plants that healers use in their treatments. But Ayensu concedes that the magic may have a beneficial psychological effect on some patients, explaining that in many of these societies the herbalists and witch doctors also serve as psychiatrists and counselors. "If that works with them," says Ayensu, "then that's fine. But my major interest rests with the chemistry of these medicinal plants."

More than half the world's plants are thought to have medicinal powers. These plants are complex chemical factories, whose active ingredients may be present in the roots, stem, bark, leaves or flowers. Most herbal medicines are mixtures, rather than single plants or plant parts. The plant acorus calamus, for instance, is currently used in fifty-one different drug preparations because its rhizomes (root stems) contain an essential oil with insecticidal and sedative properties.

The prime source of medicinal plants are the angiosperms (seed-bearing plants), perhaps because they are the most common, comprising almost two-thirds of the plant kingdom. The tropics yield the richest harvest of medicinal plants, not only because a greater number of species flourish there, but because plants from regions with hot climates are richer in active constituents than those from colder regions.

The most important medicinal constituents in plants are the alkaloids. Alkaloids are complex nitrogenous compounds that, even in small amounts, produce profound effects on the human nervous and circulatory systems. Each plant may contain fifteen to twenty different alkaloids. The amount of active ingredients in a plant is highly variable and depends on whether or not the plant was grown under favorable conditions.

Early physicians were never quite sure of appropriate drug dosages because they were unable to establish the limit between a dose that cured and one that killed. It was not until the beginning of the eighteenth century, when a German chemist, named Friedrich Serturner, succeeded in isolating alkaloids, that correct dosages could be estimated. He was the first to crystallize the morphine alkaloid from the opium poppy. In rapid succession, the active alkaloids of numerous medicinal plants were then discovered.

Plants have benefited drug research in many ways. Sometimes the constituents isolated from plants are used directly to make drugs: digitoxin comes from foxglove, morphine from opium poppies and atropine from belladonna. At other times, plant constituents serve only as the starting material for the synthesis of useful drugs: synthetic penicillin is obtained from natural penicillin, and steroid hormones are normally synthesized from plant sapogenins. Then again, there are times when the active ingredients in plants serve only as models in the making of drugs either because of the toxicity of the natural ingredient or its side effects. It was a model of cocaine, an alkaloid obtained from coca leaves, not cocaine itself, that eventually led to the development of modern local anesthetics.

Yet there is a tendency for drug companies to downplay the importance of plants in the creation of new drugs. "Most of the drugs derived from plants that are currently in use were discovered before the 1930s," says John Adams, vice-president of the Pharmaceutical Manufacturers Association. "I can think of only two new ones: the anti-cancer drug derived from periwinkle and the steroids obtained from the Mexican yam and used in the making of oral contraceptives. But for the most part, drugs are no longer derived from plant materials, and there is no major effort currently underway among American companies to screen plants."

Even the National Institutes of Health recently discontinued its plant-screening effort to discover new anti-cancer drugs. But many scientists who thought the effort was promising are very critical of this decision, calling it extraordinarily shortsighted. "It has actually cost very little money compared to the hundreds of millions of dollars that have been spent on other projects," says one highly respected chemist.

The whole thrust of drug research in America changed in the 1950s and 1960s from seeking the active principles of plants to the design of molecules through organic chemistry. The pharmaceutical industry now uses what it believes to be more "biorational" approaches such as genetic engineering and endocrinology in the development of new drugs. "One of the problems of the plant-screening process," explains Adams, "is that very often the extracts of active plant ingredients are too toxic to be used medicinally. In other cases, they are simply not potent enough to really be considered useful in the treatment of disease."

Quite apart from problems of toxicity, however, are the commercial considerations. Most American drug companies now see plant materials research as being too expensive, considering the low probability of coming up with new prototype molecules that are necessary in the development of new drugs. "When an American drug company does look into plants," says Ayensu, "they usually just hone down on one and spend a lot of money just to make sure that the FDA is satisfied before they can use it." Some natural-product advocates blame the poor results of the industry's plant-screening programs on the fact that traditional healers are not involved.

This lack of interest on the part of American drug companies is not shared by their counterparts in Europe and in other parts of the world. One plant currently attracting a lot of interest among pharmacologists in Africa and Asia, is the fagara plant, which is used as a chewing stick in West Africa. "It turns out," says Ayensu, "that fagara contains certain alkaloids that are very important for slowing down a common blood disease that affects a lot of blacks, sickle-cell anemia. The juice in it seems to unsickle. Chemists are now hard at work trying to isolate the active material."

Many other plants are currently being tested for their medicinal powers. In Britain, studies are in progress to test the ability of primrose oil (literally oil from the primrose plant) to work against eczema, multiple sclerosis, hyperactivity in children and some cardiovascular problems. The oil is already considered an effective treatment for hangovers and menstrual discomfort. Research on forskolin, an extract from a relative to the mint family herbs, is focusing on the treatment of glaucoma, which afflicts more than two million Americans over age thirty-five. When applied directly to the eye, the substance decreases intraocular pressure by reducing the flow of fluid into the eye.

Isao Kubo, a professor of natural products chemistry at the University of California, Berkeley, recently reported having found a potential source of new antibiotic drugs in some East African plants. Maesanin, which is extracted from the orange berries of the Myrsinaceae bush, seems to work against the bacteria responsible for cholera, meningitis and many infections contracted during surgery and childbirth. Maesanin may also hold clues for treating asthma. The other plant extract reported on by Kubo is polygodial, which comes from a type of smartweed known as Polygonum hydropiper. This compound seems to significantly increase the effects of a variety of antibiotic drugs in treating yeast infections.

Perhaps the most important factor leading to the recent surge of interest in plants that heal is the news of China's success in using herbal medicines side by side with modern medicine as part of its comprehensive health-care program. The news has spurred numerous scientists, foreign drug companies, and public health experts at the World Health Organization (WHO) into taking a second look at the age-old treatments and methods of the herbalists.

Because medicinal plants continue to play such a major role in providing the health needs of most of the world's people, the WHO resolved several years ago to promote a coordinated approach between traditional and modern medicine in order to achieve its goal of bringing adequate health care to all the world's people by the year 2000. The WHO realized that their goal could never be achieved by using western physicians alone, as there would never be enough of them, and so decided to enlist the help of traditional healers to accomplish this goal.

The WHO now recognizes the value of the traditional healer's experience with medicinal plants and encourages them to receive training in the ways of modern medicine. At the same time WHO is encouraging more western doctors to study the work of traditional healers and to analyze the properties of the herbs they use. The WHO hopes to be able to breed professionalism into herbal medicine by applying scientific criteria to questions of use and dosage.

"The idea," says Ayensu, "is to try to get the western-trained doctors to work hand in glove with the traditional herbalists. This is a much wiser way of approaching the whole health-care delivery system than trying to replace it. Western medicine will of course play a major role in the area of the operating theater, but in the day-to-day problems, traditional medicine will continue to keep people in good repair."

Just how traditional herbalists came to learn the appropriate medical uses of plants is not known in any great detail. Botanists reason that since throughout history humans have made use of the plants and animals that have surrounded them, they no doubt experimented with the vegetation by placing it into their mouths. In so doing they probably discovered that many plants provided nourishment, that others were toxic and that still others seemed to relieve the symptoms of sickness. From such trial-and-error experiments, certain plants may have come to be venerated for their healing properties, despite any real knowledge of how or why they had such power.

Ayensu believes that traditional herbalists may have used the doctrine of signatures as a guide in determining which plants to use on the various parts of the body. The doctrine, which has no scientific basis, holds that "like cures like." Therefore, a leaf shaped like the human heart is best suited for curing heart ailments; a plant with a milky sap is good for stimulating lactation; the walnut, looking as it does like the human brain, is appropriate medicine for head injuries; and so on. Regardless of how their knowledge was acquired, however, systems of traditional pharmacology eventually developed over the centuries and were passed on orally from generation to generation.

"It is important that we respect these herbalists," says Ayensu, citing as an example the systematic, three-year training program of herbalists in Ghana. First, an intense discipline is instilled in the students. It even requires celibacy to assure their total concentration. The students are first taken into the forest, where they begin to study the plants and their uses. During this time they also are taught to observe carefully the behavior of animals in the forest; sick or injured animals know which vegetal products to use for their ills, and the herbalists are taught to transfer this knowledge to the care of their patients. A wolf bitten by a snake, for instance, will dig up the roots of bistort, which acts as a purge and rids the animal of the toxin.

The apprentice in herbal medicine also learns to pick plants at times of their maximum potency. "Only recently have we begun to learn in scientific terms just how important harvest times can be," says Ayensu. "We now know, for example, that in certain plants alkaloid levels are low at noon and high in the evening. So what we have ascribed to magic over the years, now turns out to have a scientific basis. If we are honest we should be ashamed. We are beginning to understand that we don't know it all."

Ayensu fears that many medicinal plants and the knowledge about them may soon be lost forever. He deplores the fact that many traditional cultures have abandoned their herbal remedies for western medicines in the wake of the contact with western civilizations. And he rails against pharmaceutical companies who resell to developing countries drugs derived from medicinal plants that are readily available in those countries.

"They get the plants for literally nothing and then send the drugs back in a bottle and charge the moon for it," he says. "I think that a certain amount of equity is important here. You shouldn't have to pay for the drugs when the plants are all around."

Just as alarming, he points out, is the problem of depletion. Because the bulk of the plants used in preparing drugs are collected from the wild, the heavy collection pressures on certain plants for the many local and foreign pharmaceutical markets are causing serious shortages. Compounding this grave situation is that approximately twenty thousand flowering plant species are threatened with extinction because of cutting and burning of tropical forests and development. The loss of these plants leads Ayensu and other conservationists to wonder just how many potential wonder drugs may now be lost to us forever.

KILLER AMOEBA

Plunging into a nearby lake on a hot summer day may be one of childhood's most exhilarating moments, but for a few unlucky swimmers every year the memory of that watery adventure is short-lived. For beneath the refreshing waters, the lily pads suspended on slender green stalks, the upraised logs and past the schools of fish lurks an unexpected hazard: a tiny, nasty strain of amoeba that attacks and kills swimmers by feasting on their brain cells.

Though millions of people swim unscathed every year, the medical histories of those who have encountered these pernicious, freshwater organisms are less than comforting. Typical is the story of a fourteen-year-old boy who was admitted to a central Florida hospital several years ago in a feverish, lethargic and disoriented state. The boy had been in perfect health until two days earlier, when he had begun complaining of increasingly severe headaches. Attending physicians decided to check his spinal fluid for the presence of pathogenic amoebas after learning that he had been swimming in a freshwater lake. The test was positive and extensive treatments were begun immediately. But the boy's condition deteriorated rapidly; in just eighteen hours the boy went from an agitated state to total unresponsiveness. On the fifth day, he died.

No voodoo curse administered in some far away land or particularly malevolent deity can be held responsible for this unusually hellish episode. Instead, the culprit was nothing more than a little blob of protoplasm long regarded as a mere biological curiosity but now known to be a virulent form of free-living amoebas. First observed under a microscope in 1755, free-living amoebas (so-called for their ability to handle themselves under almost any condition) live in nature in great profusion and are usually harmless. Not until 1965 were some strains of free-living amoebas recognized to be human pathogens.

Though encounters with these amoebas are rare, more than 175 fatalities have been attributed to them worldwide, according to Dr. A. Julio Martinez, a professor of pathology at the University of Pittsburgh School of Medicine. The two most recent cases come from Texas in 1984. In Virginia, eighteen deaths have been attributed to them in the past, and in Florida, nine. There have also been victims in South Carolina, Georgia, Mississippi, Louisiana, Arizona, Utah, California, Pennsylvania and New York. No continent, no latitude has been spared. Deaths from these amoebas have been reported from Japan to Australia, from India to Nigeria and from Peru to Great Britain.

The culprit in most of the fatal infections is an amoeba known as *Naegleria fowleri*. Its victims are usually healthy, young individuals who had been swimming. They develop severe headaches, accompanied by fever, nausea and lethargy, which signals the onset of a disease called Primary Amoebic Meningoencephalitis, or PAM. Death strikes within five to seven days of infection. That quickness, combined with its flu-like symptoms and similarity to meningitis, disturbs those in the medical profession who are aware of the disease.

Still, medical accounts describing the course of the disease remain strictly dispassionate. The *Naegleria* apparently invades the central nervous system through the nasal passageway, where it attacks the olfactory nerves and enters the protective layers of the brain and the cerebral cortex. There it devours brain tissue, probably through the production of enzymes that dissolve the tissue for ingestion. The brain then swells through the accumulation of fluids, and the skull becomes very tight. Thereafter, the patient lapses into a coma and dies. Autopsies show that the victim's brain has become as soft as jelly and full of hemorrhage.

"It's a dramatic death," says Dr. Flora Wellings, director of the Epidemiology Research Center in Tampa, Florida. "And it's a dramatic disease. Children do not normally complain of headaches. Yet they will complain of a headache so severe that they won't even want you to talk to them. This is a clue."

The organism is a "bad actor," says Dr. George Healy of the Centers for Disease Control (CDC) in Atlanta. What could be meaner, he asks, "than to pick on young kids who are fond of life, swimming and having a good time? It scares me, and people who work with it have a great deal of respect for it."

There are also indications that *Naegleria* may cause infections other than through the inhalation of water. In Nigeria, several years ago, three individuals showing no prior history of swimming came down with PAM. They appear to have been infected during the windy season with *Naegleria* cysts in airborne dust. Two other children, who were found to have *Naegleria* in their nasal passages, manifested upper respiratory infections but not signs of PAM. These two lived.

Responsible for a smaller number of amoebic-related deaths are several *Acanthamoeba* strains. *Acanthamoeba* is an opportunistic organism, meaning that it takes advantage of the lowered resistance of the host. Its victims are usually the elderly, the chronically ill or those under immunosuppressive therapy, either cancer patients who have been under treatment with chemotherapy and radiotherapy or transplant patients receiving drugs to avoid rejection.

Acanthamoeba infections are generally not fatal, however. Scientists are uncertain about how *Acanthamoeba* enter the human body, but it seems to have an affinity for the respiratory tract, injury sites on the skin, the nose and especially the eyes. Recently, several cases of *Acanthamoeba* causing eye infections have occurred in the United States. Symptoms include eye irritation, inflammation and redness, as well as intense pain. These complaints can last for months, and if not treated can lead to the loss of an eye. The fatal form of *Acanthamoeba* disease is known as Granulomatous Amoebic Encephalitis, and is characterized by fever, seizures, visual hallucinations and mental abnormalities.

To date, no satisfactory treatment has been found for either amoebic disease. Both *Naegleria* and *Acanthamoeba* are remarkably resistant to a variety of drugs. Only three individuals are known to have recovered from *Naegleria*-related infections, and only one drug, Amphotericin B, has shown potential as a life-restoring agent in such cases. Few agents appear to have any effect on *Acanthamoeba.*

Scientists are puzzled not only by the potency of the organisms and their resistance to drugs, but by their erratic occurrence as well. Why some people swim in the water unharmed and others swim in the same place and get sick remains a mystery. Scientists believe that many factors may be involved in contracting amoebic infections. High concentrations of the organism in the water might play a part, though it is known that in the laboratory only one amoeba is needed to kill a mouse.

Infection may also depend on the state of the body at the time of the encounter. It is possible that some people are able to mount a better defense against the organism than others; they may, in other words, have a certain amount of natural immunity to those infections. "Since they are so ubiquitous in nature," says Dr. Richard Duma, chairman of the infectious disease division at the Medical College of Virginia in Richmond, "man probably comes in contact with them fairly frequently. So it is not inconceivable that we do get natural infections, minor ones from which we get immunity." Recent studies confirm this notion.

One factor is impressive, however, in determining the risk of infection. It appears that people taking the greatest risk are those who swim along the bottom of the water, stirring up the sediments where these organisms reside in greater concentrations and possibly in more virulent form.

Invariably these killer amoebas can be isolated from waters with above-average temperatures. They thrive in temperatures ninety-eight degrees and beyond. Not surprisingly, therefore, the season for amoebic infections in the United States occurs in late June, July and August. Artificially-heated lakes, such as those receiving thermal discharges from cooling plants, are also known to facilitate the growth of these pathogenic amoebas.

"If you look hard enough," says Dr. Govinda Visvesvara, a research microbiologist running the CDC's international registry of pathogenic amoeba cases, "you can find these organisms almost anywhere." They have been found in freshwater lakes and streams, hot springs, man-made lakes, sewage sludge, thermally-polluted canals and lakes, indoor swimming pools with insufficient chlorination and in a naturally heated, drinking water pipeline in Australia years ago. But it is still not known why certain bodies of water allow the proliferation of the organisms and other bodies of water with comparable temperatures do not.

The key may be found in factors other than water temperature. There is evidence that increased populations of bacteria enhance the proliferation of pathogenic *Naegleria*. Pollution, therefore, may be playing a major role in the population densities of these killer amoebas. Dr. Barry Commoner, director of the Center for the Biology of Natural Systems in St. Louis, believes that pollution causes a breakdown in the natural integrity of the ecosystem and may well be responsible for these amoebic infections.

"It seems likely," Commoner explains in his book *The Closing Circle*, "that in organically-polluted streams and ponds there may be enough bacteria to activate the amoebic cysts, as they enter the water from the soil where they are plentiful. Feeding on the bacteria, the amoebas then reproduce in the water, becoming sufficiently concentrated to invade successfully the brain of the unlucky swimmer." Commoner thinks that in the next thirty years, as more rivers and lakes become unnaturally burdened with organic matter, these pathogens may reproduce in such quantities as to make human infection far more likely than ever before.

The notion that these amoebic diseases have only recently begun to appear as a result of environmental pollution runs into serious trouble, however, when we consider that amoebic-related cases, diagnosed in retrospect, date back as far as 1909. The disease may actually be an ancient scourge. "People have probably been dying of it for hundreds of years," says CDC's Healy. "I think it's something that's been going on since the time when those amoebas and man met in some pristine swamp long, long ago."

Though amoebic-related fatalities are not currently on the increase, the medical community is divided on the magnitude of the public-health problem involved. Most believe that in terms of the number of fatalities, pathogenic amoebas really don't constitute a very important health problem. You're more likely to get bitten by an alligator or struck by lightning, they point out. But some believe it could become a problem in the future. "I think that as we get more and more thermal enrichment from power plants and other industries utilizing water for cooling purposes," says Duma, "that we are going to run into a sizeable amount of trouble. Besides, since it's there you can't just push it under the rug. It certainly kills a lot more people than rabies—and there are all kinds of rabies programs throughout the country."

For the most part public health measures taken in response to these pathogenic amoebas have been minimal. They seem only to be triggered by common-cause epidemics, epidemics in which several people have become infected from the same source. After an indoor swimming pool in Czechoslovakia was proved to be the source of amoebic infections involving sixteen fatalities over a six-year period, the cracked walls of the pool where the amoebas proliferated were entirely rebuilt. No amoebic infections have been reported there since. In California, after two cases (one fatal) were traced to a hot spring in the San Bernadino National Park, signs were posted warning bathers that swimming there posed a danger to their health. (But a nudist group kept tearing them down, believing it was a federal plot to keep them from bathing in the nude.)

The most dramatic public health action to date, however, took place in Richmond, Virginia, where a lake that was thought to be a major source of Virginia's eighteen fatal infections was closed by court order through the public health department. No cases have been reported in Virginia since then. Other common-cause epidemics have also taken place in Australia, New Zealand, Belgium and Great Britain.

There is no arguing that the solutions to the problem posed by these pathogenic amoebas are generally unrealistic or unwieldly. "You can't close down every lake to swimming," says Wellings. "You can't chlorinate all the lakes."

Scientists agree that the situation deserves increased attention. At the Centers for Disease Control efforts are geared toward finding ways of diagnosing the infection as quickly as possible and finding the optimal growth medium for the amoebas in order to test candidate drugs that might kill them. Other researchers are trying to discover something about the organism that would render it susceptible to containment. Wellings hopes that a natural predator will be found in lakes that don't have the deadly organism; the predator could then be introduced into contaminated lakes.

The story of these killer amoebas should not prevent you from going swimming again. It hasn't stopped the scientists who are on intimate terms with the microorganism from taking an occasional dip. Besides, if you remain truly frightened, it may comfort you to know that there are preventative measures you can take. First, use a noseguard or plugs if you are going to swim on the bottom. And make certain that when you come out of the water you blow your nose. That's right, just give the old honker a good toot.

ELECTRONIC DOCTORS

In the beginning its creators called it DIALOG. With improvements, it became INTERNIST. Now, perhaps in deference to its almost mythical powers, they have renamed it CADUCEUS, after Hermes' winged, serpent-entwined staff, the traditional symbol of the medical profession. But physicians who have made the acquaintance of this computer program designed to function like a human physician use a nickname. Half in admiration, half in jest, they call the software SUPERDOC. The latest offspring of the marriage between medicine and computer science, the new CADUCEUS is perhaps the perfect symbol of health care to come.

CADUCEUS is very much like a human expert in internal medicine, only better. Physicians today suffer from a serious case of information overload. Estimates of the number of facts required to practice internal medicine run to a million—two million if all the information used in the medical subspecialties is included. No physician can have at his fingertips all the data from such an extensive and quickly changing field. But CADUCEUS can.

A physician with access to the system feeds the patient's medical history into the computer terminal, along with the results of the physical examination and the laboratory findings. Then, with great speed and considerable accuracy, CADUCEUS sifts through its knowledge of nearly six hundred diseases and four thousand manifestations of disease (symptoms, physical signs, lab data) to arrive at a diagnosis. When the diagnostic performance of CADUCEUS' predecessor,

INTERNIST-1, was compared with that of physicians who had cared for the patients at Massachusetts General Hospital in 1969, the program proved roughly as proficient as its human counterparts in diagnosing diseases for which it had been programmed.

But CADUCEUS is not yet ready for the hospital ward. There are huge areas of medicine that the program knows nothing about; CADUCEUS still has a lot to learn. For the moment, its developers consider it experimental. According to Jack Myers, of the University of Pittsburgh's Decision Systems Laboratory, it may take up to a decade before the system is perfected and most physicians gain access to the program.

Even in its current form, however, CADUCEUS has aroused the consternation of many physicians who see the system as a prospective threat to their careers. But Myers assures them that this diagnostic tool was designed to aid, not replace, them. "I think CADUCEUS will make internal medicine more exciting," he says. Myers believes it will free physicians from their increasingly time-consuming role as mental file cabinets, and allow them more time to observe, interact with and care for their patients.

For the past couple of decades physicians and computer scientists have been laboring together to create such computer-based, medical decision-making systems. Though CADUCEUS is clearly the most ambitious application of computer science to the problems of medical diagnosis thus far, it is by no means the only one. Other expert systems, as they are known, with more limited ranges of expertise, are being used as teaching devices and research tools. At Stanford University, a program called MYCIN can select antibiotics to be used in treating bacterial infections. John Gage, of the State University of New York at Stony Brook, is developing a minimal artificial intelligence program to aid his fellow anesthesiologists. The program provides detailed information about appropriate anesthetic techniques for pediatric surgery. The system will be portable enough to be used in the operating room.

Diagnostic computer programs rely on a variety of "thinking" techniques to provide advice. MYCIN and most other computer-assisted, medical decision-making systems use rule-based inference. That is, the medical knowledge is represented in the program as a set of rules. For example, "if the whites of the patient's eyes are yellow, then he has a buildup of bile pigments in his body." The computer's inference mechanism applies each rule to reach conclusions about a patient's case. Among MYCIN's computerized colleagues are rule-based systems focusing on the diagnosis and treatment of glaucoma, the interpretation of physiological signals monitored in intensive care units and the prediction of drug interactions.

A second group of these electronic medical consultants uses a technique called statistical pattern classification. For such programs, knowledge is represented as a set of probabilities, and the computer provides the physician with the probability that each possible diagnosis is correct. One such system, which diagnoses the cause of acute abdominal pain (like that occurring in appendicitis), has already proven a boon to good patient care. In a trial conducted in Great Britain, it was found that had the computer's predictions been used rather than the physician's, fewer unnecessary operations would have taken place and fewer cases of appendicitis would have been delayed before surgery. Other systems that rely on the statistical approach have been used to diagnose congenital heart disease and to identify patients most likely to attempt suicide.

A third variation on diagnostic computer design makes use of the program's ability to compare a new patient to patients about whom data is already stored in the computer's memory. Systems using such data-base comparisons are particularly well suited to problems involving prognosis estimation, a frequent practice in assessing patients with lung cancer or coronary heart disease. These systems can also provide medical research with enormous amounts of highly-prized raw data.

But by far the most sophisticated approach to the creation of computer-based-medical decision systems involves the construction of cognitive models, programs that attempt to mimic the reasoning processes that occur in the mind of the physician. The computer conceives of an image of the whole patient, based on the disease manifestations present. It then postulates the presence of one or more maladies that could explain these manifestations and, if necessary, asks more questions in order to narrow the diagnosis. The new and improved CADUCEUS will be one such system; others include PIP, which focuses on excessive fluid accumulation in body tissues and CENTAUR, used to interpret pulmonary-function tests.

These are but a few of the many approaches being taken to create computer-assisted, medical decision-making systems. No one system is best. "Every one has very serious limitations," says medical computing expert Dr. James Reggia, of the University of Maryland's Department of Neurology. "But there are situations in which each approach can be appropriate." The important thing to remember, as studies have shown, is that the particular diagnostic strategy used by physicians, or their electronic counterparts, is of secondary importance to the associative memory of the needed medical facts.

If only for their immense capacity for manipulating vast amounts of medical facts, computers have much to offer the clinician. Yet computer technology has been remarkably slow to break into the medical profession. In most hospitals, computers are still only used for processing of patient admissions and business-office billing. Gradually, however, as the practice of medicine is viewed more and more as a problem in information management, computerized medical information systems serving both clinical and administrative needs are finding their way into hospitals across the country. They are reducing the number of lost and incorrectly identified laboratory specimens, providing more rapid interpretation and wider dissemination of electrocardiogram results and increasing the efficacy, accuracy and appropriateness of drug dispensing in the pharmacy.

One such medical support system, now in operation at the LDS Hospital in Salt Lake City, is called HELP. It contains a profile of every patient in the 550-bed hospital, making it easier for physicians and nurses to follow their progress. By acting as the physician's watchdog, HELP can reduce many of the most common oversights in medical practice. When a treatment is ordered, for instance, HELP checks to make sure that the suggested drug or test is safe for that particular patient. If there is potential trouble, the computer sounds the alert.

One of the earliest applications of computer-based patient management occurred in the field of mental health and involved the interviewing of patients by computer. Computers administer psychological tests, such as the Minnesota Multi-

Phasic Personality Inventory (MMPI), and interpret the answers in a fraction of the time and at a fraction of the cost that it would take a psychologist. To interpret the MMPI, for example, a psychologist would have to refer to thousands of references from the current psychological literature. No expert can remember them all, but a computer can. Today, more than a hundred such systems are in operation in hospitals and psychiatric offices across the United States.

Recently, other subspecialties have gotten into the act. A system is being developed in which elective surgical patients will be given a pre-anesthesia interview at a computer terminal at the time they are admitted to the hospital. The questioning lasts twenty minutes, during which dozens of yes and no questions relating to the patient's medical history appear on the screen. The resultant patient history is added to the patient's file, and the interview results are printed out for the anesthesiologist, who can then meet the patient and probe further into potential problem areas.

Though computers have a reputation for being cold and unfeeling, most physicians have found that patients enjoy their computer interview experience. Patients feel like they are in control—and the computer is always patient and polite. Many patients, in fact, feel more comfortable with the computer than with their physician. For these reasons, computers may soon be helping mental health professionals in the actual treatment of patients. Programs at the University of Wisconsin's Psychiatric Computing Laboratory at Madison are now being evaluated for their ability to provide therapy to depressed patients and assist them in adhering to their drug regimens.

The biggest barrier to full implementation of computers in medicine is, surprisingly, not computer technology but the current state of medicine itself. Physicians trying to translate their medical knowledge into computer languages have found the task stupefyingly difficult. Why? Because while computers demand an explicit presentation of knowledge, medical-knowledge language is often inherently imprecise, lacking accurate terms, definitions and a crisp, logical organization. For the computer scientist, it's like trying to turn a sow's ear into a silk purse. "We'll have good medical computing," says Dr. Donald Lindberg of the Information Science Group at the University of

Missouri, "only when we have a good understanding of medicine."

More important, some physicians fear that a computer program is not flexible enough to deal with the quirks and the unexpected turns of patient care. How can an expert system with its timeless framework of propositions and syllogisms hope to handle properly the changing biochemical cocktail known as the human body? Might not such systems become giant freezers that solidify our medical procedures and perceptions? Are not medical students being swamped by science and technology at the expense of the basic healing skills?

But the more familiar doctors are with computers, the less they seem to share in these worries. They realize that these systems are designed to serve them by relieving them of the burden of data collection and calculation, so that they may devote more time to careful patient observation and proper judgment. Though there is resistance to overcome, physician and computer expert James Reggia thinks that "Two decades from now, this technology will be taken for granted." One day its influence may even surpass the impact of Laennec's stethoscope and Roentgen's X-rays.

HOSPITAL HAZARDS

Each year, as many as ten million Americans entering a hospital with one ailment acquire another simply as a result of being there. In one study, a team of doctors found that one out of every three patients at the Boston University Medical Center, a first class institution in terms of quality health care, developed a complication during their stay as a result of a diagnostic or therapeutic procedure. These complications may have contributed in part to the deaths of fifteen patients—an average of one death for every fifty hospitalizations. On a nationwide scale, that could translate to as many as half a million fatalities a year. Public-health officials estimate that such adverse patient care costs Americans more than a billion extra health dollars each year.

In the eyes of some observers, the specter of medical mishaps in hospitals looms so large that these bastions of life and hope begin to seem more like modern-day chambers of horror. "A hospital is like a war. You should try your best to stay out of it," writes Dr. Robert Mendelsohn, a practicing physician for twenty-five years and formerly chairman of the Illinois Medical Examining Committee, in *Confessions of a Medical Heretic*. Of the estimated twenty thousand medical malpractice suits filed in the U.S. courts each year, more than three-quarters involve injuries that allegedly occurred in a hospital, according to Dr. James Cooper, of the University of Kentucky Medical School.

Physicians know well the risks of medical treatment, although, for obvious reasons, these are not generally discussed. Illnesses and complications resulting from a diagnostic procedure or a form of therapy are known as *iatrogenic* illnesses, from the Greek meaning *inadvertently produced by the physician.* But to lessen the sting of the terminology, and because so few such illnesses are actually produced by physicians themselves, many medical practitioners have come to prefer the term *nosocomial,* meaning *hospital acquired.*

The most common nosocomial illness is an adverse reaction to a drug, which accounts for about half of all iatrogenic complications. The more serious drug-related problems are serious alterations in heartbeat, abnormally low blood pressure and dramatic changes in mental states. Falls from hospital beds are much less frequent, but not uncommon. Inappropriate treatment because of inaccurate lab tests is also known to occur. In addition each year, patients are injured by anesthetic explosions in the operating room, and others are shocked or electrocuted by electrical apparatus.

Surgical errors, though rare, are frequently fatal. In a survey of patients at Boston's Brigham and Women's Hospital, a team of physicians headed by Dr. Nathan Couch found that "surgical misadventures" occurred in about one percent of the general surgical patients. For these unlucky patients, the adverse outcomes also meant an average of forty extra days in the hospital and another $40,000 added to their hospital bill. The misadventures often involved surgeons who were too quick to operate, too confident of their skills or too concerned with performing currently fashionable procedures.

Of all the medical hazards a patient may encounter in a hospital, however, infections are most frequent. More hospital patients are laid low by hospital-acquired infections each year than by heart attacks, some two million patients, according to one estimate. On the average, nosocomial infection will increase the length of a hospital stay by one week and add about $700 to the patient's bill. These infections are responsible for more deaths than any other single iatrogenic illness, more than 300,000 each year.

"The area of hospital-acquired infection hasn't captivated the American interest," says Dr. Robert Haley, "but it's definitely a serious problem." Haley is a former director of the hospital infections program at the Centers for Disease Control (CDC) and a leading expert on infection control.

Hospital epidemiologists estimate that as many as half of all nosocomial infections are preventable, and for this reason the medical community has placed a greater emphasis on controlling infections than on any other iatrogenic complication. A 50 percent reduction in the infection rate would mean a savings of over a billion dollars in health care a year. More significantly, however, if the infection rate were cut in half, 150,000 fewer people would lose their lives each year.

By definition, nosocomial infections are those that develop after the patient's first seventy-two hours in the hospital. At least 90 percent of these infections are bacterial in origin. The rest result primarily from viruses. Parasites represent a small fraction of the problem. Most are related to the medical devices that are used to treat patients. For instance, the same intravenous lines that deliver nutrients or drugs to the bloodstream can also be conduits for dangerous bacteria.

Bloodstream infections can be extremely serious. "About fifty thousand patients die each year in U.S. hospitals as a direct result of hospital-acquired bloodstream infections," says Dr. Richard Wenzel, the director of Virginia's statewide infection-control program. "That's as many as are killed in highway accidents across the nation during the year."

Hospital-acquired pneumonias are also often deadly. "Operations are the most common cause of pneumonia in hospitals," says Haley, "and these infections may often be preventable by giving the patients preoperative breathing instructions." Improper breathing can cause parts of the lungs to become stagnant and provide an area for germ growth.

Medical records show that patients undergoing surgery run three times the risk of developing an infection than nonsurgical patients do. The type of surgery being performed is a crucial factor. You are more likely to get an infection from a colon operation when the bowel is full of organisms, explains Wenzel, than from a hernia operation.

The most significant correctable determinant of the risk of surgical-wound infection, however, appears to be the surgeon's technique. Studies now reveal that if surgeons are shown their own surgical infection rates, these rates drop by half. In view of the sensitivity of such data, however, postoperative surgical-wound surveillance and reporting systems are still uncommon in U.S. hospitals.

Poor hospital design and engineering may also be contributing to the risk of infection in hospitals. Some patient-care areas, such as the nursery, which houses highly susceptible young patients close together, and wide-open, intensive-care units, which allow hospital personnel to go from one patient to another without washing their hands at a convenient sink, can play a direct role in the transmission of disease. Inadequate maintenance and housekeeping play important roles as well. The hemodialysis unit, for instance, exposes susceptible patients and personnel to kidney machines that are often difficult to decontaminate.

Although it may come as some surprise, many of the troublesome bacteria that enter the hospital enter on the patient's own body. Patients may become susceptible to these bacteria when taking steroid drugs, which suppress the immune system, or when the organisms are transmitted to a vulnerable portion of the patient's body through some diagnostic or therapeutic procedure. "Half of the patients pick up a new organism in the hospital," says Wenzel, "and in about a quarter of these cases it is possible that some of these organisms are transmitted on the hands of medical personnel." For this reason, the single most important procedure for the prevention of nosocomial infections is simply washing the hands.

Until recently, infection control was not a primary public-health issue. What sparked the interest of the medical community was a pandemic of staphylococcal disease that swept this country and other parts of the world in the late 1950s and early 1960s.

By the mid-1960s, however, the staph problem suddenly abated. No one knows why. "It came and went sort of like an 'Andromeda strain,'" says Haley. But the staph pandemic aroused everyone's awareness. Gradually, the medical community began to think in broader terms than staph, and by 1963, when the CDC held its second conference on the subject, it was no longer known as the Conference on Staph Diseases in Hospitals, but as the National Conference on Institutionally Acquired Infections.

The late 1950s were also a time of mounting fear of germ warfare, and these fears worked in concert with the staph pandemic to generate increasing concern over infections. A third force that led to the medical community's interest began in

Great Britain in the mid-1950s. There, a hospital hired a nurse (or sister, as the British call them) to be a full-time controller of infection. It was the nurse's job to roam the hospital and determine where the breaks in technique were occurring. The idea fell on fertile ground and, by the mid-1960s, had sprung up in two U.S. hospitals. The CDC soon began to recommend vigorously that hospitals do surveillance and have an infection-control nurse for 250-bed hospitals.

During the past decade, a major infection-control movement emerged in the United States. National guidelines, published and disseminated to hospitals across the country, now recommend a host of preventive measures, including a change in intravenous needles every three days, closed systems of urinary drainage, preoperative breathing instructions and a change of the breathing circuits on respirators every twenty-four hours.

While almost all hospitals have some kind of infection-control program, the one established in Virginia is regarded by the CDC as a model statewide program. It started with funding from the CDC in 1974, and its director is its founder, Dr. Wenzel, a professor of medicine and the hospital epidemiologist at the University of Virginia Medical Center in Charlottesville. Three-quarters of the state's hospitals participate in this program, in which medical personnel, usually nurses, take a two-week course on infection control. The nurses all learn how to use patient records to look for evidence of infection.

A majority of the nation's hospitals do have surveillance, but in Virginia the high-risk patients are watched most closely. As a result, only sixteen person-hours per week are needed to survey a 660-bed hospital. The program, which costs about $70,000 a year, is 82 to 94 percent accurate in reporting infections and is highly cost effective.

"If I can reduce the infection rate in the state just one-tenth of one percent," says Wenzel, "the savings would be on the order of a half to a million dollars. If I can knock it down a whole percentage point, we might save as much as ten million dollars a year in Virginia alone."

As might be expected, surveillance data on hospital-related problems have caused some nervousness in the medical community. Some doctors and hospital officials feel that the collection of such data may offer patients increased opportunities to bring medical malpractice lawsuits. Without these data, however, infection control cannot succeed. Wenzel manages to assuage the fears of hospitals by arguing that the data document the hospitals' efforts to maintain vigilance and reduce risk and are therefore generally helpful both medically and legally. A national survey of hospital administrators seems to bear him out. Nearly all hospital administrators believe that surveillance data are not a hindrance to defending the hospital against litigation for alleged malpractice, and more than half believe that the information is helpful to their case.

Although hospitalization is still hazardous, most people would argue that the benefits far exceed the risks. But that was not always the case. It was not until the early 1900s, according to Harvard medical historian and biochemist Lawrence Henderson, that patients began to have a better than even chance of being helped by doctors. Nowadays, the medical community is making a concerted effort to develop further monitoring mechanisms to assess and reduce all the hazards of hospitalization and patient care. Luckily for us, they have already come a long way.

HEART BALLOON

It was on the day Frank Sinatra was in town, Joseph Skripek remembers, that an X-ray picture of his heart revealed a severe blockage in his right coronary artery. Two weeks before he had begun feeling severe chest pains, the most common symptom of heart disease. "I was virtually disabled," recalls the forty-five-year-old attorney from Wayne, New Jersey. "I couldn't walk a block without feeling the pain."

Until recently, heart-bypass surgery would have been his only hope. But now, Skripek learned, he had a choice. His alternative was a relatively new procedure that seems at first glance almost child-like in its simplicity. The procedure, known as coronary angioplasty, involves inserting into the artery a tiny balloon on a plastic tube that is gently inflated at the site of the blockage to open the arterial passage.

Being only mildly sedated, Skripek was able to watch the entire process on the same monitor the cardiologist used to guide the tiny tube, or catheter, to the site of the blockage. "You see the tube running around in your heart," says Skripek, "and you watch to find out if the doctors are going to succeed. It's almost like cheering on your own team. But when you win, you win big."

Skripek won big. He was back at work within a couple of days. But he is clearly one of the lucky ones. Each year more than a million Americans lose their battle with heart disease, the number one killer in the United States. Basically, heart disease (of which coronary artery disease or atherosclerosis is by far the most common type) occurs when not enough blood gets to the heart muscle. This is caused by a narrowing or blockage of the arteries leading to the heart. No one knows why this occurs, though doctors suspect that cholesterol and smoking have something to do with it.

Until the late 1960s, when heart-bypass surgery was introduced, there were few ways for heart disease victims to get relief from pain. Under attack for overuse lately, the bypass eliminates the symptoms by increasing the supply of blood to the heart. Medicines only reduce the workload on the heart, and thus its demand for oxygen, by making it beat more slowly and with less force. But the patient must change his way of life.

Compared with the heart bypass, a grim and awesome series of surgeries, coronary angioplasty is something of a minor miracle. In a bypass, the patient has general anesthesia, then the surgeon removes a portion of a vein from his leg, cracks open the chest and grafts the vein around the area of obstruction. After the operation there is a two-week hospitalization and a long recovery at home. In contrast, the patient undergoing coronary angioplasty feels only slight discomfort while under local anethesia and can usually resume his daily activities within a few days.

"Coronary angioplasty represents the first major change in the treatment of this very prevalent disease in more than a decade," says Dr. Dennis Reison, the director of the coronary angioplasty program at Columbia-Presbyterian Medical Center in New York City. He estimates that nearly a quarter of all patients with coronary-artery disease can now be successfully treated with angioplasty instead of bypass surgery. This alternative means a considerable savings in health-care costs; while a heart bypass runs upward of $25,000, a coronary angioplasty costs only about $5,000.

Tawny, blue-eyed and baldish at the age of thirty-four, Reison has performed more than 150 coronary angioplasties since he established his program in December 1982. The procedure is also available in many hospitals throughout the country. It is estimated that some fifty thousand coronary angioplasties will be performed in the United States this year.

While neither this technique nor bypass surgery is a cure for heart disease, both are quite effective in eliminating the illness's major symptom, chest pain. Studies published in *The*

American Journal of Cardiology show that coronary angioplasty increases the blood flow to the heart in three-quarters of
all patients. The other quarter repeat the procedure after a
year. "Unlike bypass surgery," says Reison, "angioplasty can
be done again and again with no additional risk."

Yet coronary angioplasty is not a panacea. Patients with
many lesions in lots of vessels are still best served with bypass
surgery. Reison, whose father is now ill with atherosclerosis,
knows this all too well. "He had an angiogram," says Reison,
referring to a procedure in which dye is injected into the arteries to identify blockages, "and it showed too many lesions in
multiple vessels to use angioplasty. He's going to need a
bypass."

"It bothers me that he is ill," Reison continues, "not only because I love him very much but also because I know there is a
genetic predisposition for the disease. I am presumably at a
higher risk to develop it myself." Thus, Reison exercises regularly, stays on a low-cholesterol diet and doesn't smoke. He
had no knowledge of his father's illness when he chose to be a
cardiologist.

Reison, who grew up on Long Island and went to Yale and
Stanford Medical School, chose to specialize in angioplasty, he
explains, "because I'm aggressive and action-oriented. Like
other angiographers, I'm probably a frustrated surgeon. But I
didn't want to be a surgeon because of the long hours, the mili-
tary-type training and the strict attitude it requires. Medicine
is much more of an intellectual challenge."

Reison learned coronary angioplasty at Emory University
from Dr. Andreas Gruentzig, a German cardiologist who originated the technique in 1977. But angioplasty (*angio* meaning
vessel, *plasty* meaning plastic or changeable) actually dates
back to 1964, when two American physicians, Charles Dotter
and Melvin Judkins, began using progressively larger catheters to open blocked leg arteries. By the early 1970s, European
physicians began applying the same technique to the narrowing of arteries in the kidneys.

It was Gruentzig, however, who refined the procedure for the
kidneys by using a balloon-tipped catheter instead of progressively larger catheters. Once he had miniaturized the kidney
balloon and developed the technique and equipment, he per-

formed the first angioplasty on a human coronary artery in September 1977. But the practice did not become widespread until a few years later when the technology had improved still further.

The turning point was the introduction of the steerable catheter. Inside this new catheter is a wire with a thin platinum tip. Easily bent, the wire allows the cardiologist to make small steering changes through the maze of coronary vessels. "The new wires work so that if you make half a turn at one end you get half a turn at the other end," Reison explains. "To achieve the same turn with the old catheter, you had to turn it four or five times, like power steering, and you were never quite sure of the result on the other end. In this business, you don't want power steering."

In a typical procedure, a catheter is inserted into a vein in the patient's neck and brought down into the heart to a plane just above and perpendicular to the blockage. This catheter marks the area of obstruction on the cardiologist's monitor. Then a pre-formed guiding catheter is inserted into an artery at the groin, pushed up through the aorta, which is the body's major blood vessel, and fitted into the opening of the artery that feeds the heart muscle. A smaller balloon-tipped (dilatation) catheter then fits inside the guiding catheter.

Next, the cardiologist positions the balloon so it straddles the blockage, and he inflates it several times, each inflation lasting thirty to ninety seconds. Afterward, he measures the pressure on each side of the blockage, injects some dye to see if the blocked artery has opened up, and when satisfied with the result, removes the catheters.

The procedure lasts from about one hour, for an easily accessible lesion in one vessel, to about three hours, when there are lesions in several vessels. Reison has done as many as seven lesions at one time. He sees no limit to how many lesions can be treated this way in a patient, "as long as the blood vessel is not totally closed and the blockages are reachable by catheter."

Just how angioplasty works is not completely understood. "This debris that narrows the arterial passage is a combination of cholesterol, calcium and blood clot," Reison explains. "It doesn't really get squished into the walls of the artery when the balloon expands, because it's too hard. We think what happens is that it fractures and reforms. Then after a while, the body takes up this deposit." But the deposit doesn't simply get washed away. It's the structure of the artery itself that's damaged. These blockages are a disease of the entire vessel.

About one percent of the patients who undergo coronary angioplasty die from it. "The major risk is that the vessel is going to block off," says Reison, "that it will clot in the area of the blockage. If that occurs, then no blood flow gets to that artery, and a heart attack occurs. We always have an operating room and a surgeon ready to do a bypass in case something does go wrong. This happens in about 5-to-10 percent of the cases in the national experience, but ours has been much less than that."

Reison expects that within five years (when the technology has been refined and the expertise is available at all community hospitals) the procedure will be the treatment of choice for nearly half of all coronary-artery-disease patients. This number includes many patients who previously used only medications because bypass surgery was too risky for them. It also includes more than a tenth of each year's 250,000 bypass patients who have a recurrence of symptoms within the first year and for whom the risk of a second bypass is much greater.

Skripek, for one, is thankful to have bypassed the bypass. "The only thing going through my mind during the procedure," he says, "was the fear that if it didn't work I'd be cracked open like a lobster. As soon as I realized they had opened up the artery, I felt incredible relief."

NEW VISION

Diana Stokke has always been extremely nearsighted. "My parents would take me for drives in the country as a child," she recalls. "They would point out a particularly colorful bird in a tree, and I would say, 'What tree?'" An ophthalmologist later determined that she had 20/4,000 vision. A person whose vision is worse than 20/400 can no longer read the big E at the top of the eye chart. "I was absolutely helpless," says Stokke. "It's a severe handicap to be so visually impaired."

Her search for a satisfactory solution led her through the gamut of ophthalmologic remedies. She tried wearing eyeglasses, but they were very heavy and, she says, "they made people feel like they were looking at me through the wrong end of a telescope." She couldn't wear hard contact lenses at all, and she couldn't see well with soft lenses. Even extended-wear lenses, she says, "weren't without drawbacks."

Then her ophthalmologist told her that he would soon be performing a new operation, called a myopic keratomileusis, or MKM, that might solve her problem. The details of the operation made her cringe, but she decided to try it.

Stokke underwent one of the most ingenious and controversial procedures in modern eye surgery. Under local anesthesia, a section of the cornea of her right eye was sliced off, reshaped to correct for her nearsightedness, and stitched back into place. Three days later, when the ophthalmologist removed the patch from her eye, her vision in that eye had already improved to 20/50.

"It was amazing," says Stokke, a caterer and cooking teacher in her late thirties. "I could see immediately. And in the two weeks that followed I could tell on a daily basis that my eyesight was improving. It was the answer to a lifelong dream."

Stokke is one of several hundred people to have undergone the operation in the United States. It is offered by about a dozen surgeons nationwide, and Stokke's ophthalmologist, Dr. Robert Rubman, is one of the few eye surgeons currently performing the operation in the New York area. "I first learned about this procedure during my residency program," says the thirty-nine-year-old ophthalmologist, a graduate of New York University School of Medicine. "I thought it was exciting beyond belief."

Stokke's operation is one of several new procedures in the rapidly growing field of refractive eye surgery. By changing the shape of the cornea so that the light coming into the eye is properly focused on the retina, refractive surgery can correct near-sightedness, farsightedness and astigmatism without the need for glasses or contact lenses.

Rubman, who is himself slightly myopic, thinks that this type of surgery could potentially benefit many of those who wear glasses or contacts, some 30 percent of the population by his estimate. Of his own contact lenses, he says: "I can function without them. But if I weren't happy with them, I would entertain the possibility of having refractive surgery."

Of all the new refractive procedures, perhaps the most controversial is radial keratotomy. RK, as it is known, corrects for myopia by flattening the curvature of the central portion of the cornea. Tried first in Japan in the 1930s and refined in the Soviet Union in the 1970s, RK in its current form generally involves making eight equidistant radial incisions in the cornea beginning about three millimeters from the corneal center. The depth of the incision varies from 80-to-95 percent of the corneal thickness. Too shallow an incision produces no change in visual acuity; too deep a cut perforates the eye. Today, hundreds of surgeons offer RKs, and thousands have been performed in the United States since the procedure was introduced here, in 1978.

"But 'miracle' surgeons are giving this procedure a bad name," says Rubman. "It's being spearheaded by a bunch of buccaneers who are touting it as a cure-all. It's not. RKs work best for those with low myopia. The older you are and the less correction you need, the more successful RKs tend to be. The younger you are and the more nearsighted you are, the less successful you'll be with an RK, because when you're young the white part of the eye is easily deformable, and the cornea may not flatten where you need it the most."

Extremely nearsighted people would probably benefit more from MKM, the operation that Diana underwent, says Rubman. The genius behind this procedure is Dr. Jose Barraquer, an eye surgeon in Bogota, Colombia, who spent twenty years developing the instruments and perfecting the procedure. Rubman learned the operation from Dr. Lee Nordan, a San Diego ophthalmologist who studied with Barraquer.

The technique involves slicing off about 60-to-70 percent of the central portion of the cornea with a cutting tool known as a microkeratome. The sliced corneal disc is then transferred onto a $70,000 machine called a cryolathe, which freezes the tissue, rotates it and allows the surgeon to carve in the patient's prescription.

"All the adjustments (the curvature of the arc that the tool describes, how far you go into the tissue) have all been determined by computer," says Rubman, who unabashedly revels in modern ophthalmology's new technology. He spent five months practicing on the cryolathe with some sixty donor corneas before performing his first operation in the fall of 1983. "All I have to do," he continues, "is feed in the patient's corneal curvature, the thickness of the section and how much we want to correct. Everything else is taken care of." Once the correction has been made, the tissue is thawed out and sewn back on the patient's eye. The fifty-four-step procedure is performed under local anesthesia and takes about ninety minutes.

"It's like making a living contact lens out of the patient's own cornea," says Rubman. "It's really exciting to be able to rehabilitate the eye in this way, to free someone of glasses." But it's only within the last couple of years that the cryolathe has become reliable enough for interested ophthalmologists to undertake this procedure with confidence. The major turning point was the introduction of digital monitors. Accurate to one-thousandth of a millimeter, the readouts now give the surgeon the precise location of his cutting tool as it shaves the corneal disc.

A similar refractive procedure corrects farsightedness.

Hypermetropic keratomileusis, or HKM, is utilized by some surgeons to treat farsightedness in patients whose previous eye surgery precludes an implant or contact lens. The procedure involves shaving the patient's own corneal disc in such a way that when it is sewn back on the eye the center of the cornea bulges out slightly. Advocates of the procedure claim it produces better, quicker results with fewer complications than two rival operations, both of which involve donor corneas.

Several refractive techniques are also available to control astigmatism. Again, a new one known as the Ruiz procedure is preferred by some ophthalmologists to two of the field's oldest workhorses, the corneal wedge resection and the corneal relaxing incision. The challenger attempts to control astigmatism by making two trapezoid-shaped incisions and three horizontal cuts on the cornea's steepest meridian.

No one can guarantee that these new refractive procedures will result in perfect vision. "But we are fairly certain that we can get a patient to see 20/40 or better," says Rubman, who is on the staffs of Mount Sinai Medical Center and Manhattan Eye, Ear and Throat Hospital. "We are aiming for driving vision without correction. So far, our results have been even better than that. All these procedures can be fine-tuned; they can be repeated. That's the nice thing about them." While patients may notice improvements as soon as the eye patch comes off, exactly how much each individual's vision will improve is impossible to determine until several weeks or months have passed.

Despite its promise, refractive eye surgery is not for everyone. First, it cannot correct presbyopia, the difficulty that older people have seeing up close; second, it cannot be performed on diseased corneas; and third, it cannot improve on a person's best corrected vision. "If your potential was only 20/50 before the operation, you will only be able to see 20/50 afterwards," says Rubman. "But if the potential is there for 20/20, there is an excellent chance that you will see in the 20/20 range afterwards.

"In my practice, 4-to-5 percent of the patients are unhappy contact-lens wearers, or at least lenses didn't fulfill their expectation," says Rubman. "These people are good candidates for refractive surgery."

Sometimes refractive surgery may be the only workable solution to a problem that neither glasses nor contacts can correct. Some jobs (police officers, fire fighters and flight attendants, for instance) require a certain level of vision without glasses. "It can open up occupations and sports that were formerly closed to many people," says Rubman. "And even when the operation appears to be simply cosmetic, by allowing people to be free of wearing glasses, it can actually open up whole new dimensions in their personality."

The major issue for those considering refractive surgery is likely to be the expense involved. While eyeglasses run anywhere from $80 to $200 and contacts cost up to $600, the going rate for an RK or a Ruiz is about $2,000 for each eye, and MKMs and HKMs are about $3,500 for each eye. While a few insurance companies will cover these procedures, some will make only a "contribution," and others refuse to cover them at all.

Considering the money involved, the skills and equipment necessary to perform these operations, and the enthusiasm that some ophthalmologists have shown for doing them, it is no wonder that the subject has been a matter of considerable controversy. Those who offer these operations are either applauded by colleagues for their courage and innovation or accused of overenthusiasm for still unproven procedures.

The more conservative ophthalmologists think that most of the problems being treated by refractive surgery are better handled with glasses and contacts. They are alarmed by the recent surge of interest in these procedures. They worry that their colleagues are operating on too many patients too soon without the benefit of long-term follow-up studies. They are concerned about possible eye damage or loss as a result of complications during or after surgery. They question whether the promised benefits outweigh the considerable costs.

"The procedures look promising," admits Dr. D. Jackson Coleman, head of the department of ophthalmology at New York Hospital-Cornell Medical Center. "But, as surgical procedures, they are new enough and potentially dangerous enough that they need to be evaluated a great deal more before we would consider them beyond an experimental or desperate situation. The techniques are relatively safe, but the full range of complications and long-term results have not yet been established. Certainly the number of situations in which a very safe procedure, such as glasses or contact lenses, isn't satisfactory is relatively small in my opinion. I don't think that people should have these operations for cosmetic or social reasons, though they could be appropriate for people whose career goals can't otherwise be fulfilled. To me that's a relatively desperate case. But I think in general it's still too early to offer them to the public as a new breakthrough."

Rubman and the dozen or so other ophthalmologists who perform these operations insist that in the right hands these procedures are safe, sound and ethical. "There has never been an eye loss due to infection," says Rubman, "and the problem of scarring has been largely eliminated by careful technique. As the equipment has gotten more refined in the last few years the results have improved and many of the complications have been eliminated."

After weighing all the pros and cons, it is the patient who must make the final decision. "It was my sense of trust and confidence in Dr. Rubman that finally convinced me to have the operation," says Diana Stokke. Once the vision in her right eye had stabilized completely, she had the operation done on her left eye. "When anyone asks me if the operation was worth it, I say it was indeed. I think it will change people's lives."

SUDDEN DEATH

The democracy of death insures the inevitable: a reservation for the final voyage. Yet the schedule of departures is not available to all, and as a consequence the major form of mortality in the western hemisphere is that quick, frightful leap into the dark known as sudden death. Clinicians define sudden death as "rapid, unexpected, natural death afflicting seemingly healthy people." They use the terms natural to exclude accidents, homicides and suicides, and rapid to mean anything from instantaneous up to about twenty-four hours preceding the onset of death.

This catastrophic syndrome accounts for one-third of all natural deaths in the United States, the majority of which are cases of sudden cardiac failure. Normally an underlying heart disease can be found to explain cases of sudden death. But because many people with severe cardiovascular conditions live long and useful lives, some clinicians have begun to wonder whether other contributing factors are involved. They also wonder whether these same factors might not be behind the 25,000 or so cases of death each year that are not only sudden but unexplained as well.

Leading the list of causes is something that has been the focus of much medical research in recent years: intense emotions. The idea that emotions can provoke sudden death has had widespread acceptance ever since civilization began. History and folklore are full of stories about people dying in the throes of some powerful emotion. The Biblical personage Ananias died, apparently of fright, when Peter told him: "You have not lied to man but to God." History also tells us, for example, that the Roman Emperor Nerva died of anger, Pope Innocent IV succumbed to grief, King Philip V of Spain dropped dead of humiliation and one Chilon of Lacedaemon made his exit from an overdose of joy while embracing his son, who had just carried away a prize at the Olympic Games.

The idea has also enjoyed a wide credibility among physicians. Almost two thousand years ago, the Roman scholar of medicine, Celsus, wrote that emotional states could affect the heart, and in 1628 the discoverer of circulation, William Harvey, reaffirmed the observation. But the idea fell into disrepute in the late nineteenth century once the fledgling science of modern medicine declared that all causes of death could be determined at the autopsy table. The earlier notion is now being reexamined, however, as a sizeable body of evidence accumulates linking emotions to destabilized heartbeats, and ultimately, to death.

Until recently, little data have been available on the psychological states of victims at the time of their deaths. But with the advent of cardiopulmonary resuscitation techniques and improvements in emergency medical services, many people now survive serious heart attacks. This fortunate circumstance has allowed some researchers to talk to the victims and find out what their emotional states were just before the attack. In a study of 117 resuscitated patients conducted at Boston's Brigham and Women's Hospital, a fifth of the patients reported suffering from "acute emotional disturbance" just before their life-threatening arrhythmias, seriously abnormal heartbeats that can culminate in death. Among the disturbances they listed were bitter arguments, some public humiliation, marital problems, business failures, profound grief and, in one case, nightmares.

"There is strong evidence for a link between stress and sudden cardiac death," says Dr. Regis DeSilva, a cardiologist involved in the study, "but the association still lacks definitive scientific proof." The chief problem he says, is the difficulty of translating emotions like despair and fear into clinically verifiable measurements. What evidence there is does suggest that things like stress, fear, hopelessness and even the act of heavy breathing can activate the sympathetic nervous system, the part that marshals energy for instant use in the "fight or flight" response. Switching on this nervous system, doctors say, can trigger arrhythmias and cardiac arrest.

In the 1930s one celebrated doctor in India demonstrated the power of the mind and imagination in an astonishing and deadly experiment he performed on a criminal who had been condemned to death. The convict was an assassin of distinguished rank, and court permission had been obtained to bleed him to death inside prison so that his family might be spared the disgrace of a public hanging. When the time came, the condemned man was blindfolded, led into a room and strapped to a table. Under it a container was set up to drip water gently into a basin on the floor. The doctor pricked the skin of the man's arms and legs near his veins as if to bleed him and at the same time started the water dripping. The convict believed that the dripping he heard was his blood flowing out, and when the sound of the dripping water at length stopped, he passed out and died—without actually losing one drop of blood.

Of all the psychological stresses, it appears that fright is the one most likely to cause rapid and sudden death. George Engel, a psychiatrist at the University of Rochester School of Medicine, in New York, has collected 170 case histories of emotional sudden death and found that more than a quarter of them involve some "setting of personal danger or threat of injury, real or symbolic." The list includes cases of terrified patients who died just before a minor surgical procedure. Aware of this possibility, some surgeons refuse to operate on patients who fear surgery.

People can be scared to death. A team of pathologists, Marilyn Cebelin and Charles Hirsch, found that in 15 of 497 cases of assault in Cleveland between 1950 and 1979, the physical injuries the victims suffered with a variety of weapons (including a cane, a coat hanger, a belt, an electric cord and a shoe) should not have killed them. Eleven of these fifteen people had developed lesions in the heart similar to those that form in experimental animals subjected to great stress. The researchers concluded that the victims had died of fright.

A fine line separates fright from despair, however, and it is possible that some victims die of hopelessness rather than emotional shock. This seems to be the case in sudden deaths among primitive people, a phenomenon known as Voodoo Death. Forty years ago, Walter Cannon, an authority on psychosomatic medicine, searched through the records of anthropologists who had lived with primitive people in widely scattered parts of the world and found numerous reports of otherwise healthy people dying inexplicably. One case concerned a Brazilian Indian who, condemned and sentenced to die by a medicine man, found himself helpless against the pronouncement and died within a matter of hours. Another case dealt with a young African who ate a banned wild hen and who, on being discovered, was overcome by fear and died within twenty-four hours.

If there is any light at the end of this dark tunnel, it may come from one unusual group of victims whose deaths may offer some clues to exactly how these sudden cardiac deaths occur. These are the Asian refugees in this country who have been particularly susceptible to so-called nightmare deaths. They constitute the single largest category of unexplained sudden deaths yet discovered.

In just four years, some forty Laotians, Vietnamese and Kampucheans have died mysteriously in their sleep. The victims were mostly young, apparently healthy, men. Death in each case happened at night and took only a matter of minutes. This strange pattern had first been noted in the 1940s and 1950s among young men in Japan, where the disease is called *Pokkuri,* and among Filipino men in the Philippines and Hawaii, where the disease is known as *Bangungut* (the Tagalog word for nightmare). Autopsies done on the men revealed they had suffered acute cardiac failure, but none had underlying heart disease. Because some deaths were .preceded by heavy breathing, groaning and screaming, the popular notion arose that the deaths were caused by nightmares.

If doctors can find out exactly what happened among these refugees, says Dr. Roy Baron, an epidemiologist formerly of the Centers for Disease Control in Atlanta, they may well have a clue as to what caused other inexplicable sudden deaths. Cardiac pathologists who studied the heart tissue taken from people recently deceased think the heart failure may have originated from some abnormality in the heart's connective tissue, its electrical system. While that would explain why these hearts are vulnerable, it would not explain what triggered the

instability that resulted in death. Perhaps the best way to locate the trigger factor involved, Baron suggests, is to find
people who have survived these episodes and study them in
sleep laboratories.

"I don't think we are going to get very far by arguing that
these people had a bad dream and scared themselves to death,"
says Dr. Merrill Mitler, a sleep physiologist and former chief of
the Sleep Disorders Center at the State University of New York
at Stony Brook. Right now the leading hypothesis, which is not
inconsistent with the autopsy and case history material collected by Baron, Mitler says, is that REM (rapid-eye-movement)
sleep precipitates a kind of cardiovascular crisis.

For vulnerable individuals, REM sleep may be fraught with
risk. During REM the sleeper has no control over body temperature and becomes paralyzed. Try a tendon reflex during REM
and there will be no response. During wakefulness, respiration
is largely under the control of the amount of carbon dioxide in
the blood, but that is not true during REM, when the respiration becomes highly irregular. The heart rate can also become
extremely irregular during this phase of sleep. Statistics show
that heart attacks occur most commonly during the nocturnal
hours of greatest REM frequency. Some research even suggests
that the sudden death syndrome in infants happens during this
period of what is called paradoxical sleep.

"While everyone shows some cardiac irregularity during
REM sleep," Mitler asserts, "there may be a subgroup who
exhibit terrific cardiac irregularities during REM. What we
would like to do is study that subgroup in which these night
deaths are most frequent and see whether we can find any
exaggeration of normal cardiac and respiratory irregularities."

Studies like Mitler's may eventually help pinpoint some of
the high-risk factors. But at the moment a mountain of medical
uncertainty separates risk factors from a knowledge of actual
causes. The crucial question remains: What causes the fuse to
blow?

UNIVERSE

STAR OF ENLIGHTENMENT

Perhaps the most remarkable archeological find of the century is an old clay tablet that contains a record of stellar observations dating back to the dawn of human civilization. The tablet—so small that it fits in the palm of the hand—is replete with cuneiform symbols invented by the Sumerians, mankind's first-known civilization. The tiny tablet is believed to be a temple scribe's miniature copy of an ancient catalogue of stars, constellations and astral deities. Though the tablet itself may not be much more than three thousand years old, the text appears to reflect aspects of astronomical knowledge dating back nearly six thousand years. Cuneiform scholars refer to the tablet as BM-86378, a regrettably drab designation in view of the startling clue it holds to the most spellbinding episode of celestial pyrotechnics ever recorded by man.

On a section of the tablet that can be covered by a small-size postage stamp, among references to Capricorn, Sagittarius and Scorpius, there is mention of a giant star in a region of the heavens where no prominent star was known to exist until quite recently. According to George Michanowsky, a linguist and specialist in Mesopotamian astronomy, Sumerian legend holds that this mysterious star was deified and held responsible for the blossoming of their civilization. The tablet locates this great star in an area of the southern sky where the constellation Vela meets southern Puppis. To cuneiform scholars in 1912, when the tablet first came to the attention of the scientific community, the reference was puzzling but did not appear all that important.

But within this narrow celestial region, an Australian radio telescope pinpointed, on October 4, 1968, a drastically shrunken, fast-spinning neutron star, which astronomers call a pulsar. The pulsar is now known to be the collapsed remnant of a supernova. PSR 0833-45, as the pulsar is currently catalogued, emerged from a gigantic cataclysm that occurred long ago in the far southern constellation Vela. Astrophysicists refer to this particular supernova as Vela X. Nine years after its discovery, astronomers finally managed to pick up optical flashes from the pulsar. It was, they said, "the faintest thing ever seen."

At one time, however, the Vela star in its supernova stage was magnificently visible to the naked eye. Astronomers now recognize it as the nearest and brightest known to science. The pulsar it left behind is located thirteen hundred light-years from our solar system, less than half as far away as the second nearest supernova, which appeared in the constellation Lupus in A.D. 1006. And it's three to four times closer than the Crab Nebula, a product of the celebrated A.D. 1054 supernova in the constellation Taurus.

The Vela X spectacle probably appeared most startling to the early inhabitants of southern Mesopotamia, now part of modern Iraq. From their unique vantage point just off the Persian Gulf, these people were able to witness a dazzling ball of light just above their southern watery horizon. When visible at night, it shone brighter than the full moon, its luminous reflections on the waters of the Gulf extending like a shiny ribbon all the way to the shore. When visible during the day, it was so bright that the starburst resembled a small "second sun" low in the southern sky. After many months, this "guest star" faded away, but not without having had a profound influence on its observers in this part of the world.

Within centuries of the appearance of Vela X, these ancient Mesopotamians, the Sumerians, developed into the earliest civilization of which we have any record. They were responsible for establishing the foundations of astronomy and mathematics and all the other arts basic to human development. They gave us the wheel and a law code at least 150 years older than that of the renowned Babylonian king Hammurabi, as well as the first love song, the first school system, the first parliament and the first directory of pharmaceutical substances. Just about all their great achievements can be traced to their development of the first full-fledged form of writing. It is no wonder that the distinguished scholar Samuel Noah Kramer once argued that history actually began at Sumer.

The connection between Vela X and Sumerian civilization was discovered by George Michanowsky. Born in Yalta in 1920 and a United States citizen for over forty years, Michanowsky is an independent scholar of many interests. He is well versed in astronomy and archaeology and a host of related subdisciplines, including linguistics, epigraphy, mythology and historical geography. He contributes to various encyclopedias, acts as a consultant on aerial and satellite-borne reconnaissance and is the archives chairman and a science advisory board member of The Explorers Club in New York City. Michanowsky's discovery is recounted in his book *The Once and Future Star*.

After careful study of that very special cuneiform tablet in the British Museum, Michanowsky concluded that a giant starburst had actually been observed and recorded by the Sumerians, and that their reaction to the event set the stage for civilization as we know it. The celestial event, he argues, not only drew their attention, but stimulated their interest in astronomy and in developing records of what they saw. This idea has been called "one of the more audacious scholarly claims in many years."

Most remarkable, perhaps, is that the Sumerians associated their own quantum jump in civilization with the sudden appearance of the great star in the sky. Just how this association came about (how the supernova was perceived as responsible for the flowering of Mesopotamian civilization) can best be explained as a psychological and cultural effect. Michanowsky contends that the human capacity to be awed by such a spectacular event in nature probably led to efforts to record and explain its appearance. Certainly the psychological impact of this celestial phenomenon was overwhelming.

Vela X must have been the "talk of the town." Writing about Michanowsky's discovery, Columbia University psychiatrist David Forrest stated in the July 1978 issue of the *Journal of Biological Psychology* that such a major celestial event "would focus the attention of everyone in unison throughout the area of earth from which it was best visible." Storytelling would no doubt have received a great boost and may well have culminated in the invention of writing. Significantly, the very first and most fundamental symbol in Sumerian script was a star.

The event, Michanowsky believes, served as "a cultural organizing principle." It was one of those electrifying moments when human knowledge took a dramatic leap forward. Explains Forrest: "Many of the empirical concepts of modern science may have had their philosophic and psychologic ancestry in Vela X. The limited play of Vela X's light upon a small sector of the horizon might have suggested the concept of focal and specific action or agency in the early Sumerians, a concept conducive to realism, progress and science, in contrast to passivity and fatalism."

The deification and mythic process surrounding the starburst was probably facilitated by the appearance of the shining star at such a low level in the sky. Says Forrest: "Man could look the phenomenon in the eye and conceive of a deity at eye level, like a friend and helper of equal status, rather than one to whom he would only look upward in awe and fear." The concept of deity incarnate would be advanced and with it the seeds of religious and divine intervention.

The heavenly event actually became the source of many of our creation myths, cosmological concepts and cultural traditions, according to Michanowsky. The date of creation as reckoned by many religious traditions hovers around 4,000 B.C., a date in tune with current astrophysical estimates of the age of the Vela supernova. Michanowsky even suggests that the interest in the heavens Vela triggered in our ancestors was so powerful that Vela may be responsible for the "deep-down feeling" so many people have that humanity is intimately bound up with the stars.

There has also been speculation regarding what physical and biological effects the supernova may have had on Earth and life upon it. Scientists have suggested that cosmic rays unleashed by the explosion of a supernova in the "solar neighborhood" could have a considerable impact on the terrestrial environment. It seems likely that a "nearby" supernova could shower the Earth with enough radiation to have produced significant mutations in terrestrial life. Vela X, though quite near, is somewhat outside this hypothetical solar neighborhood. But among all the so-called young supernovas, it is the best candidate for earthly effects, according to NASA scientist John Brandt.

Michanowsky's quest for accounts of supernova observations in ancient scripts and rock carvings spans more than a quarter of a century. Early on, he believes he may have found references in the tribal mythology of the Andes and the Amazon to what eventually became known as the Vela supernova. Later, however, he became convinced that the most promising avenue for evidence of ancient observations of Vela X had to be undertaken among the records from Mesopotamia, the so-called cradle of civilization and the region where religious traditions place the Garden of Eden. His research led to that tiny clay tablet in the British Museum and to his discovery that the tablet not only mentioned the giant starburst but also provided its precise location in the heavens. Recently, he has been able to corroborate the Sumerian accounts with references to that formidably influential star in Egyptian hieroglyphs and the glyph writing of the ancient Maya.

Michanowsky's evidence is compelling. He found that Sumerian legend tells of a giant star in the southern sky that was held sacred to the god Ea (also known as Enki). Most noteworthy among all the references to Ea is that line on the small clay tablet that reads: "The gigantic star of the god Ea in the constellation Vela of the god Ea." The subsequent line on the tablet places this great star just south of the star Zeta Puppis, the precise location of the Vela pulsar.

Ea was known as the god of wisdom and as the ruler of the southern ocean and the heavens above it. He was also the local deity of the ancient seat of Sumerian culture, the city of Eridu (now Abu Shahrain), to which the northernmost waters of the Persian Gulf once extended. Ea's Eridu and Vela both appear in a meaningful sentence found on another tablet: "The Eridu star, the star of wisdom."

A symbolic account of the Vela starburst and its influence on civilization comes from the priest-historian named Berosus who wrote an early, Greek language history of Mesopotamia at about the time of Alexander the Great. His chronicle recounts the tale of Oannes, a creature half-man and half-fish, who is described as having emerged from the Persian Gulf to teach the early inhabitants of Mesopotamia the arts of civilization. Berosus describes Oannes as giving man "an insight into letters, and sciences and every kind of art."

Astronomers, such as Carl Sagan, have suggested that the legend could be explained in terms of a possible visit by an extraterrestrial being who might be responsible for the rise of Mesopotamian civilization. But Michanowsky believes otherwise. He thinks the Oannes legend actually owes its origin to the Vela star. He explains that in time mythology would transform the star's role into that of a god teaching humanity the arts of writing and mathematics. The deity would quite likely be perceived and remembered as a human form walking on the water toward the coastal inhabitants. Its approach by a water route may have suggested to them its fishlike characteristics. It is worth noting also that Oannes is actually a Hellenized rendering of the name Ea, who also happens to be referred to in some Mesopotamian texts as the "fish of heaven."

Michanowsky has also uncovered evidence of an ancient Egyptian tradition surrounding the spectacular Vela star. One tantalizing link to the supernova is the Egyptian goddess Seshat, who strikingly resembles the Sumerian wisdom goddess Nidaba, a star-related deity and a female counterpart of Ea. Seshat was regarded as the goddess of numbers and measurements, as well as the patroness of scribes and architects. She was usually pictured holding a writing instrument in her hand. "Sesh" means write in ancient Egyptian.

Michanowsky soon began to suspect that Seshat was the Egyptian personification of the Vela star. One clue came from a tomb inscription, translated decades ago by the eminent Egyptologist Sir Alan Gardiner, that mysteriously states: "Heaven is pregnant with the Seshat star, heaven brings forth the Seshat star." Other clues confirmed his suspicions. Seshat's home was believed to be at the foot of the cosmic tree in the far-southern sky. She was usually depicted with a seven-pointed star affixed to her head by a vertical stem. This became her hieroglyphic symbol, despite the fact that stars in ancient Egypt were consistently five-pointed. The seven-pointed star, on the other hand, is a Mesopotamian phenomenon. This fits well with the notion, conceded by many scholars, that there was a Sumerian influence on the early stages of Egyptian civilization.

Seshat's curious head ornament resembles the Sumerian's cosmic tree, the seven-fronded palm tree. And it is worth noting here that one of the cuneiform components of the Sumerian name for Vela was derived from a stylized drawing of the sacred palm tree. There is even speculation among scholars that the tree of knowledge mentioned in Genesis was originally the palm of southern Mesopotamia.

Perhaps the most intriguing Egyptian link to ancient Sumerian lore about the starburst is the fabled looped cross, the Ankh, which was the Nile country's symbol of life and is presently in vogue worldwide as a good luck charm. Michanowsky was thrilled to find that Seshat was often referred to in hieroglyphic texts as "mistress of the House of Ankh." The discovery led him to conclude that the Ankh symbol is actually a stylized representation of the Vela starburst. The loop at the top of the Ankh, he states, represents the actual starburst, the horizontal line symbolizes the southern horizon, and the vertical bottom line stands for the reflection the star cast in the water. Three planetariums, including the prestigious Hayden Planetarium, have incorporated Michanowsky's visualization of "Ankh as Vela starburst" in their star shows.

Michanowsky continues to uncover evidence that links the origins of civilization to the appearance of that special star in the southern sky. The most recent development is his discovery of a Maya connection for the Vela supernova. Recent excavations in Central America indicate that the Maya civilization began much further back in time than originally estimated. The glyph writing of the Maya is still largely undeciphered; only numerical, calendrical concepts and a few "dynastic" sequences having been read thus far. But Michanowsky says he has now deciphered a mysterious glyph complex on a Maya stela as an ages-old tradition about the observation of the Vela supernova. He also relates it to the famous so-called Zero Date of the Maya, a sacred calendrical number that signified the beginning of the "current" era of the Maya world.

Reactions from scholars to Michanowsky's daring thesis have been wide-ranging. He has attracted both critics and supporters. Among the critics is E. C. Krupp, the director of the Griffith Observatory in Los Angeles. "I have no doubt that the supernova occurred," says Krupp. "I have no doubt that it was observed. But I don't think its impact is what he says it was—

that the supernova went off, stimulated people and that civilization took off from there."

Among Michanowsky's supporters is the curator in charge of the Ancient Near East Department at the Metropolitan Museum in New York. Vaughn Crawford has confirmed Michanowsky's readings of the cuneiform passages that form the basis of his work. Crawford states that Michanowsky has "conducted a scholarly and wide-ranging study of scientific sources," and that his investigative method has been "highly conscientious throughout." Michanowsky's astronomy seems equally impeccable. Richard Stothers of NASA's Institute for Space Studies in New York reports that "the results of my astrophysical investigation of the Vela pulsar strongly support the validity of [his] decipherment of ancient astronomical passages."

Work in astrophysics has actually confirmed that the Vela pulsar occurred within the time period indicated by Michanowsky's archaeological findings. According to Stothers, who is also an historian of astronomy, the newly established margin for the Vela pulsar's age falls between five thousand and eight thousand years ago. "The object may therefore be of historical significance," he stated in the April 1980 issue of the *Publications of the Astronomical Society of the Pacific*. On the basis of Michanowsky's discovery and within his newly-established margin, Stothers thus places the most likely age of the Vela pulsar at about six thousand years. Support for Michanowsky also comes from one of the world's foremost pulsar experts, Columbia University's David J. Helfand. He said that "neither the radio, optical nor X-ray observations are inconsistent with a pulsar birth around six thousand years ago."

Michanowsky's scholarly reconstruction of the Vela event is clearly one of the most revolutionary astroarchaeological speculations advanced in recent decades. His work has transformed the Vela starburst from an object of purely astronomical interest to one of considerable historical significance. At the very least, his quasi-poetic insight has caused a whole generation of specialists to think across disciplinary frontiers. If he is correct, then Vela may well be the most important star in human history. The most important star, Michanowsky points out, next to the sun.

FIRE FROM HEAVEN

During the early 1970s, a young biologist conducted an experiment in the basement of the Stanford Medical School that set the stage for a bold new theory concerning the sun's influence on the Earth and human behavior. It began with a routine study of cardiac stimulations on chick embryo hearts, organs so small (two millimeters long and a half millimeter wide) that they had to be anchored with human hairs. The setting, with its strain gauges, flowing solutions and bubbling test tubes, looked for all the world like the lab of a mad scientist. But the scientist in this case, named Marsha Adams, was far from mad. Even today, after her theory has drawn the flies of contention from the scientific community, she is viewed as a top-notch scientist whose integrity, sincerity and dedication command the respect of supporters and critics alike.

Once the study of cardiac stimulants was completed, Adams took the results to the American Heart Association (AHA), which encouraged a presentation based on the effects of the stimulants. But then suddenly, just a few weeks before the AHA presentation, the results that Adams had promised to discuss reversed themselves. Instead of stimulation, the chick embryo hearts began exhibiting depression. Assuming the experimental setup was at fault, Adams dismantled the entire system, changed the platinum electrodes, the stock solutions and the air tanks. But no matter what she did, she couldn't replicate her results.

Soon after, though, for no apparent reason, the experiment began to work again. After several of these reversals she called in her supervisor to troubleshoot the system, but he too was at a loss to explain what was happening. Having taken into account humidity, temperature and all the other factors that biologists usually control in their experiments, Adams was left with only one conclusion: "The chick embryo results were a clue that something in the environment was profoundly influencing biological processes, but at the time I didn't know where to look for it."

Intrigued by this and other instances of biological variability that had occurred during her career, Adams left Stanford to become the research director of the Women's Community Clinic in San Jose, where she collected and studied a very large data base of biological variability. The data base consisted of some eleven thousand cases of measured surgical bleeding. She noticed that the measurements of blood loss varied, and decided to screen the cases against a variety of factors in the geophysical environment, including cosmic radiation, several measures of geomagnetic and solar activity, as well as a number of standard weather variables like barometric pressure, temperature and relative humidity. Much to her surprise, she found that the bleeding anomalies occurred following periods of increased solar activity and preceding large-magnitude earthquakes.

When she brought her data to the attention of the clinic staff, she expected derision. Adams was surprised. "They said they could have told me that because everything goes haywire around there a few days before an earthquake," she recalls. "People in the recovery room showed an increase in the number of people vomiting and reacting to anesthetics. They didn't have to look at the data to tell when an earthquake was coming. When I challenged them to predict the next earthquake, they did, and the bleeding data showed the expected anomalies."

It then dawned on Adams that humans might be valuable tools in forecasting earthquakes. And why not? After all, why shouldn't human beings be as sensitive to seismic activity as the animal population has been shown to be by the Chinese? Wouldn't it be easier, she thought, to gather such information from humans, who can monitor themselves, rather than from animals, who require constant twenty-four-hour-a-day observation?

So in 1978, when Adams moved to a position as senior systems analyst at SRI International, a nonprofit California think tank, she began a study using human subjects to forecast earthquakes. Her only contact with most of the sixty people who came to participate in the study was over the telephone and she took great pains, in the interest of scientific objectivity, for them not to know one another.

Many of these volunteer subjects contacted Adams after recognizing that many of their own flu-like symptoms seemed to precede large-magnitude earthquakes. One caller told Adams: "You are my last hope before seeing a psychiatrist." Another said: "I really feel weird about this, but you've heard about those Chinese studies with animals responding to earthquakes, haven't you? Well, I think maybe that happens with people, too." They would then go on to describe the symptoms they felt before an earthquake, none of which their physicians could tie to specific illnesses.

Among the sixty individuals who reliably exhibit physiological sensations prior to a quake—"responsives" Adams calls them—are a doctor, an engineer, an interior decorator, a few nurses and a couple of secretaries. Twice a day they fill out a chart, noting the presence or absence of such symptoms as fatigue, vertigo, chills, headaches, nausea, a ringing in the ears or a flushed sensation. The form also provides a space for depression and for fights with a spouse or workmates.

Once the symptoms reach a peak of intensity, the responsives call in to a hotline set up by Adams and give their name, date, time of day, symptom and its strength. This allowed her to establish a track record for each person that shows her how accurate he or she is with regard to large- or small-magnitude earthquakes, to local versus global quakes and to the timing of the event. One person, she reports, has called only four times, but he has been 100 percent on the mark for earthquakes over magnitude 7 on the Richter scale (8.5 is "devastating"). As a team, the responsives have been accurate 80 percent of the time in forecasting earthquakes in the San Francisco Bay area within an eight-day time frame. Adams makes no attempt to forecast all of the more than 36 earthquakes of a magnitude 6.5 or greater that occur around the world each year. All forecasts are recorded by a computer that time-stamps each entry.

"I sit up and pay attention when they call," says the forty-year-old researcher. "It's awesome to watch the system work, especially when a dozen or more subjects who haven't contacted you for weeks call within a twenty-four-hour period. It really makes you wonder what's out there, because unlike color or odor, we don't sense it directly. But there certainly is something out there precipitating all those calls."

Looking for connections among apparently disparate data, Adams has discovered something that Carl Sagan would call a "natural conspiracy." ("Science," he has observed, "might be described as paranoid thinking applied to nature.") She believes that whatever force is triggering those human somatic sensations is probably also responsible for large magnitude earthquakes and the strange behavior of animals preceding those upheavals. Her data suggest that the agent responsible for this and other assorted mischief is an increase in solar activity.

The list of factors Adams claims may be influenced by increases in solar activity is a long one and includes not only earthquakes and periodic human illnesses, but also freak weather conditions, arson, riots, political instability and crime waves. Adams points out, the Falkland Islands were invaded soon after an increase in solar activity. Also on the list are railroad derailments and accidents involving airplanes, buses and ships. All these events tend to occur in specific time slots within about a week of increases in solar activity. Human reactions normally take place within the first few of days of a solar flare and earthquakes in about four days.

"I didn't start out as a sun freak," says Adams candidly. "But I've come to realize that almost all variations that occur in biological and physical processes may be the result of fluctuations in solar activity. I have to think very hard to come up with one that isn't. I suspect that all geophysical processes, including volcanoes and weather fronts, are related to solar activity in some quite comprehensible way."

These observations strike the heart of one of science's most dramatic junctures, the influence of cosmic forces on the Earth and on human behavior. To many social and physical scientists, the notion that life on Earth may be sensitive to the convolutions of a celestial body ninety-three million miles away smacks of astrological hocus-pocus. Yet these same scientists are perfectly willing to admit that life arose in the primordial broth by the action of sunlight on simple molecules. They also agree that the sun is constantly bombarding the Earth with all manner of radiations, the effects of which we are only dimly aware. Nor would they argue the sun sustains all life on Earth. The bottom line is that many scientists are philosophically reluctant to embrace the idea that the sun can hold such an intimate relationship with human life. It seems that each branch of science prefers to regard its subject matter as a closed system, operating through feedback rather than through outside influences.

Interest in, and claims for, the sun's influence on terrestrial processes have existed for well over a century. Perhaps the most exuberant proponent of solar-terrestrial interactions was a Russian professor named Alekandr Chizhevskii, who is referred to by Soviet researchers as the "father of heliobiology." Pouring over Russian archives, Chizhevskii compiled a record of recurring social events, which he compared to fluctuations in solar activity, specifically the appearance of spots on the solar disk. He produced many studies during his lifetime (1897–1964), all of them indicating an association between solar activity and such things as wars, revolutions, migrations and epidemics of cholera, influenza, typhus, diptheria and meningitis. Chizhevskii never believed that the sun actually caused these events, only that it made these events more likely to happen.

More substantive evidence for the sun's mysterious influence on human physiology was discovered shortly before World War II by Maki Takata, a Japanese physician and professor at Toho University in Tokyo. He was known at the time for having developed a test called the Takata reaction, which is a measure of albumin in blood serum. In males, it was assumed to be constant, but in females it varied according to the menstrual cycle and was a basic analytical tool for gynecologists. But when in 1938 every hospital using the test reported a sudden rise in the albumin levels of both sexes, Takata undertook a series of experiments over the next twenty years that showed that changes in blood serum occur mainly when a major group of sunspots cross the sun's central meridian, a well-established indicator of the sun's most active phase relative to the Earth. The physician found that the reaction was inhibited during solar eclipses, as it would be when tests were performed in a mine shaft six hundred feet underground.

Soviet research tends to support the notion that our blood is directly affected by the sun. The number of lymphocytes, which normally make up about a quarter of the white blood cells in our body, have been shown to decrease during periods of intense solar activity. It has been reported that the number of diseases related to lymphocyte deficiency actually doubled during the tremendous solar storms of February 1956.

Similar studies abound. An analysis of 5,580 coal mine accidents in the Ruhr in Germany showed that most of them occurred on the day following spurts in solar activity. A study by a British epidemiology unit found a correlation between the periodicity of sunspots and the occurrence of influenza pandemics. A survey of 28,642 admissions to psychiatric hospitals in New York led to the conclusion that psychiatric disturbance shows a marked increase during periods of natural magnetic field intensity, a parameter on which the sun has a known influence.

Though the work of Marsha Adams treads on familiar ground, it would be incorrect to conclude that there is nothing new under the sun. Adams parts company with her predecessors in isolating which factors control the timing of such biological, mechanical and geological variability. To begin with, it is not sunspots, she insists, but solar flares that may be the key to solar influence.

Solar flares are the most spectacular and powerful of all forms of solar activity. These mammoth, tongue-shaped protuberances display temperatures in excess of twenty million degrees Kelvin and release the energy equivalent of ten-to-one hundred billion one-megaton H-bombs, enough power to supply the United States for thousands of years. Flares usually appear in step with the sunspot cycle, which reaches a maximum approximately every eleven years. At times of solar maximum, when the greatest number of spots appear on the sun, as many as two or three small flares may appear every hour, and one enormous flare may appear each month. But at times of solar minimum, when the active regions of the sun are not facing the Earth, weeks may pass without any significant flares.

Erupting flares unleash a tidal wave of radiation, electrical and magnetic fields and high-energy particles into space, part of which enhance what is known as the solar wind. When this solar debris smacks into the Earth's magnetic field, or magnetosphere, a wide variety of terrestrial effects occur: aurora borealis, geomagnetic storms, electrical surges in power lines and even in the ground itself. During one such outburst in 1859, telegraph operators found that they could transmit and receive messages without batteries.

"What has not been appreciated," notes Adams, "is just how much biological responsiveness there is to solar activity. Unfortunately, studies on solar-terrestrial interactions do not show a one-to-one correspondence. So one wonders if there is not some other factor that might actually be the mechanism that triggers this biological responsiveness. There is another factor that coincides with solar activity and that is ELF."

ELF is Extremely Low Frequency electromagnetic radiation (3 to 30 hertz), in other words, very long radio waves. It is produced naturally in two ways. The first is through solar activity. When the main bulk of particles shot from the sun during a solar flare finally hits the Earth's magnetic field, it rattles the magnetosphere the way a hungry chimp might shake a bread box. This flapping of the magnetosphere generates ELF. ELF is also produced indirectly through a second channel of propagation—through weather fronts.

Adams is currently testing the hypothesis that ELF might be the geophysical variable responsible for triggering all kinds of biological and seismic processes. Unfortunately, relatively little work has been done on wavelengths below 100 hertz. But biological processes are known to respond to several frequencies within this range. A somewhat casual German study of 53,000 subjects, for example, seemed to show that people take longer to respond to normal stimuli when they are in the vicinity of ELF waves. Biologists studying ELF in the lab and field have come up with a list of symptoms remarkably similar to those Adams' responsives report.

It is also known that the frequency of alpha brain waves (8 hertz) has a geological parallel in what is called the Schumann Resonance, the frequency at which the length of a radio wave equals the circumference of the Earth. This piece of information set Adams wondering whether ELF might not also help directly trigger earthquakes.

Geologists understand the action of plate tectonics perhaps better than any other aspect of seismic processes these days, but the one great mystery that remains is knowing just when one tectonic plate will break free of another and set the Earth's crust to crumbling. The key to solving that mystery lies in isolating the final nudge that upsets the balance of frictional forces locking the edges of the plates together. Adams believes that ELF may eventually prove to be that mysterious trigger. Though she doesn't claim to know just how ELF provides the final nudge that brings on the catastrophe, she does speculate on two possible mechanisms: piezoelectricity and magnetostriction.

Piezoelectricity is a process by which electromagnetic energy is converted to mechanical energy or vice versa. It occurs most notably in crystals, and it is the basis for the quartz watch. The quartz picks up the electromagnetic signal and converts it to a mechanical vibration which is then amplified. Perhaps the Earth's crust begins to vibrate through such an effect, says Adams, or through magnetostriction, a process by which certain magnetic materials change shape when they are subjected to a magnetic field. When subjected to an oscillating field, such as ELF, a mechanical motion, or vibration, is produced. Might such a mechanical vibration, set off by ELF at a frequency that resonates with a fault location that has accumulated the most strain, be sufficient to trigger an earthquake? Only further research will tell.

Though unfamiliar with the work of Marsha Adams, David Simpson of the Lamont-Doherty Geological Observatory in New York, reports that the Soviets have been somewhat successful in using low-frequency radio signals to predict earthquakes. Using a number of ground wire antennas and a standard radio receiver, the Soviets are looking for changes over time in the output of ELF, but the principle is the same. Says Simpson: "It seems to work but we don't know why."

Adams has also had some success at earthquake forecasting based solely on measurements of solar flares. She found that about a quarter of all large flares are followed by large magnitude earthquakes. Although that essentially doubles the earthquake rate one would expect by chance, it doesn't allow for very reliable forecasts. Only with accurate measurements of flare polarity and directionality could this type of forecasting succeed, she believes.

Forecasts using Adams' solar responsives as intermediaries have been more reliable. Apparently the responsives act as biological transducers and are quicker at absorbing and integrating information than any current scientific instrument. Eventually, however, Adams expects to be able to separate the human variable from the forecasts, and make daily forecasts of earthquake probabilities, like a daily weather forecast, using direct measurements of ELF and/or solar activity to supplement the human data.

Certainly the most eye-opening aspect of Adams' current forecasting system is the finding that responsives need not be in the vicinity of an earthquake in order to forecast it. Low-frequency radio waves travel around the world many times with minimum attenuation because the cavity between the Earth and the ionosphere acts as a vast natural resonator for electromagnetic energies of these wavelengths. This effect allows responsives in one locale to predict quakes anywhere in the world.

"I strongly suspect," she says, "that the information that would allow us to determine location can be found in the symptoms themselves. What seems to be happening is that even a person who has the same symptoms over and over may have additional symptoms that appear to be location dependent. For instance, I've noticed that the flushed sensation and chills seem to be prevalent for earthquakes that are to occur within a one hundred-mile radius of the San Francisco Bay. The timing of the calls may also provide location clues. Looking at track records, I've noticed that for some individuals, if the quake doesn't occur within a day of their call, the probability of the disturbance being local decreases."

Adams' forecasting system is both a byproduct of the process she describes and the means by which she hopes to prove her theory correct. "The real proof of the theory," says Adams, "is its ability to forecast." But the theory actually offers potential far beyond earthquake forecasting.

A list of potential applications might include medicine, for instance, which could reap large benefits. With an on-line computer interpreting fluctuations in geophysical variables like ELF, physicians would have at their fingertips more precise expected values for specific medical tests, which today are subject to a wide range of interpretation because of the large variability known to occur in their results. Physicians might also decide to alter a patient's drug regiment according to known geophysical correlations. These days drugs are prescribed in unit doses, but it may be that the need for those drugs varies, so that on some days a person might not need the drug at all, while on other days a doubling of the normal dose might be necessary.

Geophysical readings might also be translated into staffing needs for police and fire departments. Adams provided several fire forecasts for Andrew Casper, while he was chief of the San Francisco Fire Department. Casper had been on the track of an arsonist with more than thirty fires to his credit. "She was right on target," says Casper. "When Adams forecast, he hit within seventy-two hours. From our standpoint, she's got it down."

Psychiatry might also benefit from Adams' theory. Could it be that phases in the behavior of manic depressives are simply a response to cyclic processes in the environment? "I've received many letters from manic depressives saying how they feel that some external force is influencing their lives," says Adams. "Of course, the last thing I want to do is write back and say you are being controlled by radio waves—they would lock me up, too." But Adams wonders whether the ELF might not be producing its effects through the same mechanism held to be responsible for mood shifts in manic depressives, namely changes in serotonin and noradrenaline levels, two of the brain's natural chemical messengers of behavior. The idea came to her when she realized that the symptoms her subjects report prior to an earthquake were strikingly similar to those reported by manic depressive patients.

To explore these applications, Adams left SRI International in 1983 and formed the Time Research Institute (TRI). "What we want to do with TRI," she explains, "is look at the correlations between just about anything (human health, earthquakes, human performance, accidents, fires and explosions) and environmental changes. Right now we are collecting in real time some forty different environmental variables, including ELF, geomagnetic activity and so forth."

Not surprisingly, the theory's potential applications have played a large part in capturing the public's attention, when news of her work was first leaked to the press a few years ago. Jerry Brown, then governor of California, was intrigued enough by her earthquake project to call her, and subsequently Adams was invited to describe her work before a hearing on earthquake prediction and preparedness held by the state's Assembly Committee on Governmental Operations. The committee gave her a courteous reception and wished to be informed of further progress in her research.

The U.S. Geological Survey's (USGS) Office of Earthquake Studies in Menlo Park also gave her an opportunity to present her work, but the majority of its scientists apparently felt that the evidence she presented was not persuasive enough to warrant funding by the USGS. C. Barry Raleigh, a geophysicist with the USGS at the time, however, indicates that they encouraged her to pursue her work. California spent some $15 million that year on earthquake prediction work without any appreciable results.

Dealing with a subject of such scope involves risks, and Adams' theory has invited its share of criticism, much of it by geologists. "I never saw pulled together the kind of critical evidence required to make a hypothesis like that be even marginally acceptable," says Raleigh, now director of the Lamont-Doherty Geological Observatory, who has been outspoken in his criticism of her work. "The idea is interesting, but it was not backed up to my satisfaction by an adequate body of objective data that could allow you to decide if there was anything to it or not. Probably the weakest link in her work is that there is no reasonable physical model that might explain the phenomenon. But there is obviously something in the idea that has her convinced."

Other USGS scientists were bothered not so much by her interpretation as by the analysis of her data. "I'm puzzled by her work," says one seismologist. "There is a feeling here that her correlations are an artifact of the way she handled her figures, and that has led her astray."

But John Derr, also of the USGS, feels a Catch-22 situation

was involved in the reception of her presentation at the USGS. "The USGS seems to have adopted the position: Prove it to me and then we'll be interested," he says. "It's a standard response for proposals outside the realm of traditional science. Personally, I think Adams' work is important. It has great potential significance and definitely deserves to be pursued."

It is really not surprising that Adams' theory should stir such disbelief within parts of the scientific community because Adams felt much of that same disbelief at first. "I started out not being at all convinced," she recalls. "But I think that anyone who is exposed to the system and sees it operate very quickly loses much of their initial skepticism. I'm now quite sure that some environmental factor is having a strong influence on biological processes. Where the environmental influence is coming from is, I think, much more speculative than if it gets sensed. I might be wrong about the ELF, but that's the hypothesis I'm testing at the moment. Unfortunately, my critics often mistake for truth what I say is theory."

Adams regrets the premature publicity she has received. It has forced her to present her work through the media, without first having the results presented in a scientific journal, and even more important, without first having completed a rigorous analysis of all her data.

William Whitson, who was then director of the Governor's Task Force on Emergency Preparedness, feels he may have been partially responsible for pushing Adams beyond her own sense of scientific propriety. "I was pressing Adams to try to give us the near-term probabilities of a California earthquake based on her theory," says Whitson, an expert in strategic planning, crisis management and defense mobilization. "I did so because I feel that her theory has a lot going for it. What I find particularly interesting is the theory's predictive force and to what extent public policy could bank on it. Adams says it's just not that refined yet, but neither is any other predictive method where Earth changes are concerned."

Even in its formative stage, however, Adams is clearly excited by the theory. "Here is a variable that we are not aware of and yet is present and influencing all our lives," she says. "I think everyone may be sensitive to it to some degree. It's just that people are not aware of what to look for. It's a matter of exposure, recognition and awareness. Unfortunately, I think that right now we are culturally biased against this particular variable. People don't like to communicate their psychological and behavioral changes. Most of us don't go around saying 'I feel depressed today,' though we may occasionally report a headache. You would be surprised at the tremendous relief people feel when they sign on to the study. Some say: 'You mean it's not some psychological quirk that I have?' I've gone so far as to write excuse notes to people's bosses when they've asked me to explain their occasions of memory loss or spaceyness while at work."

While many of Adams' colleagues remain skeptical about her work, her notion that the sun has a profound effect on our lives would certainly have come as no surprise to "Uncle Joe" Cannon, the venerable Speaker of the U.S. House of Representatives between 1903 and 1911. During a debate on appropriations for solar research, it was Uncle Joe who argued: "Everything hangs upon the sun, sir, and it ought to be investigated."

SUNSTRUCK

The heavens have always held an irresistible fascination for mankind. And of all the objects in space, perhaps the most intriguing is the star closest to us, the sun. Today, high atop Mount Wilson on the outskirts of the glittering Los Angeles basin, astronomers are fulfilling the ancient quest to understand our parent star—but that isn't their primary goal. Their aim is to focus in on stars beyond the sun. In doing so, however, they are discerning remarkable details that have proved the kinship of the sun to the stars.

This unlikely approach has spawned a whole new specialty known as solar-stellar astronomy. While the bulk of the observations in this field are performed by steller astronomers, the theoretical work is done largely by solar physicists trying to get a better understanding of the sun. So this no man's land, this solar-stellar connection, as the field is known to its hundred or so practitioners, has actually been a new meeting ground for astronomers.

In the past five years, there has been a veritable explosion of knowledge in this field. Astronomers have been able to detect several sun-like features on other stars; they have found stars with sunspot cycles, stars that rotate faster at their equator than at their poles and one star whose surface vibrates with a frequency of just minutes. The new findings have come from applying what we know about the sun to other stars. But in the process astronomers have learned much about the sun itself—its erratic past, how it generates energy, how sunspots arise, and what lies in the sun's far, far future.

154

A decade ago the task of looking for solar-like features on other stars would have been an astronomical fantasy. "At that time, a lot of astronomers thought that stellar astronomy was pretty much dead," says Douglas Duncan, a young and enthusiastic stellar astronomer at Mt. Wilson. "We already knew the size, mass, composition and temperatures of stars. And there was no hope of finding the sorts of details—the freckles and warts so to speak—that solar astronomers were finding on the sun. It seemed that most of what could be gathered about stars had been gathered."

Even today, no telescope is powerful enough to let us directly see details such as sunspots, or rather starspots, on the surface of even the nearest star, certainly not the sixty-inch telescope at the Mount Wilson Observatory. In fact, this telescope, which was the world's largest at the time of its completion in 1908, is now virtually worthless for most faint object observation because of the huge sea of lights emanating from the Los Angeles basin.

What allows the astronomers there to use the sixty-inch telescope so effectively is a new technique, a unique instrument attached to the telescope that counts with great precision the number of photons, or units of light, in a particular wavelength in the spectrum of light from a star. The device, known as an HK photometer, measures the intensity of a star's light, or emission, in those parts of the spectrum known as the calcium H and K lines. These lines hold a very special significance to astronomers. Since they know that the brightness of the emission from the hot calcium gas in the sun's chromosphere, the region directly above its visible surface, is directly related to the amount of activity on the sun's surface, they have assumed that the same must be true of stars as well. By the word activity, astronomers mean flares, sunspots and the magnetic fields with which these features are associated.

Named logically enough the HK Project, this effort at Mount Wilson is being carried out by a team of more than a dozen astronomers from the United States and Europe. And because of the project's impressive results, it has been granted exclusive year-round use of the sixty-inch telescope. The honor is perhaps unique in contemporary astronomy; no other major telescope in the world is currently devoted to just one project.

Astrophysicist Andrea Dupree, director of the solar and stellar physics division at the Harvard-Smithsonian Center for Astrophysics in Cambridge, Massachusetts, sheds light on what the project means to the field of solar-stellar astronomy. "Astrophysics today is trying hard to extend what we know about the sun," she says, "by devising ways of measuring and understanding the same phenomena, the same physics, but under different conditions, in other stars. If you are a scientist, you don't just want to look at a single star like the sun, which is of a known chemical composition, known age and not terribly active, when the rest of the universe consists of stars that are hotter and cooler, younger and older and of different chemical compositions. Any scientist making a model to explain what is going on with the sun must look at stars under varying conditions to see if the model still works. It is the diversity of phenomena which tests your physics, your techniques and your ability to understand it all. And it is my personal belief that unless we really understand what is going on in the sun and the nearby stars, we won't be able to understand what is going on in galaxies or globular clusters. What are they, after all, but conglomerates of stars?"

All the stars are suns, and so any understanding of the stars must begin with an understanding of the sun, the nearest star. For millenia the sun was seen as an "unspotted perfect sphere," as Shakespeare said, but Galileo changed all that when he observed dark spots on its surface in 1610. By keeping track of them over time he calculated that the sun rotates every twenty-seven days.

Two centuries later, a German astronomer named Heinrich Schwabe noted that sunspots followed a cycle that was about eleven years long. The only known exception to this pattern occurred between 1645 and 1715, when sunspots were rare and Europe suffered a succession of unusually cold days known as the Little Ice Age. This period of solar inactivity is now known as the Maunder Minimum, after Edward Maunder, who first noted it in 1894.

Perhaps the greatest technological breakthrough in solar studies took place in 1807, when the physicist Joseph von Fraunhofer placed a card with a narrow slit on the eyepiece of his telescope, directing the sun's light through a prism. This enabled him to observe for the first time the sun's spectrum, a horizontal band of colors from red to blue. Within them were six hundred vertical lines where very little light appeared, and Fraunhofer assigned to each of the most prominent of these lines a letter, such as sodium D and calcium H and K. By 1859 the physicist Gustav Kirchhoff showed that these lines are associated with certain chemicals when they are vaporized in a flame. The following year, Anders Angstrom, the Swedish physicist, applied these findings to the sun and discovered the presence of hydrogen and other elements in the sun. His work opened the door for other scientists to study the physical nature of stars in the same way.

But few astronomers saw the promise of spectroscopy until the early part of the twentieth century. One of these visionaries was the great scientific entrepreneur George Ellery Hale, who in 1904 took two burros, a carpenter and a pair of Pasadena architects to the summit of Mt. Wilson. Hale's main interest was the sun and its physics, and it was here, on Mt. Wilson, that he wanted to erect his first solar telescope.

When Hale began observing sunspots he noticed that the patterns in the shape of the gas formations around the spots looked like the iron filings around a magnet. That suggested to him the presence of magnetic fields. Shortly afterward, he was able to confirm that sunspots were regions of very strong magnetic activity by applying the new findings of a Dutch physicist. Pieter Zeeman's experiments had shown that light in an intense magnetic field possesses spectral lines that are split into two or more components.

The discovery of magnetic fields on the sun led Hale to wonder if the thousands of stars in the same stage of evolution as the sun, but hidden to us by distance, might not also exhibit magnetic fields. He proposed to make a "study of the physical phenomena of selected stars. . .as we are now making of the sun," and even built another telescope, Mt. Wilson's sixty-inch, specifically for this purpose. But by the time it was completed astronomical interest had shifted to questions about the structure of the universe. Before long astronomers would learn that we lived in an island galaxy in a universe full of other island galaxies.

The glamour and excitement of extragalactic astronomy kept

the search for stellar analogs to solar activity on the back burner until quite recently. The first breakthrough in the field of solar-stellar astronomy came in the late 1970s with Olin Wilson's discovery of activity cycles on other stars. In March of 1966, this energetic, pipe-smoking stellar astronomer began a solo study of the calcium emissions emitted from the chromospheres of about a hundred stars in the solar neighborhood. Every month for eleven years Wilson recorded the emissions from each of these stars.

"The existence of these emission lines in stars had been known since 1912 but nobody had pursued it," says Wilson, feet propped up on his cluttered desk. Though now retired, he still comes in almost daily to the Pasadena, California, office of the Mount Wilson and Las Campanas Observatories. "I had looked into it in the late 1930s, but photographic spectroscopy is very difficult, time consuming and not as accurate as one would like, so I decided at the time that a project looking for stellar variations would have to wait for better technology."

What Wilson had been waiting for, a high resolution spectrum scanner and a highly stable electronic system for counting photons, became available in the 1960s. Shortly after it was installed on Mt. Wilson's one-hundred-inch telescope, Wilson began his groundbreaking study. "When I started out I figured I had about a one-in-four chance of finding anything," he says, "so it wasn't the kind of thing a young guy would want to place a bet on. Only some old geezer like me could take the time to sit there for more than ten years and look at these things."

Wilson's patience was well rewarded. He eventually found that many of the stars showed regular cycles in the same range as the sun's own eleven-year cycle. This discovery was of revolutionary importance for those trying to explain the solar cycle, the central problem in solar astronomy for the past century. The rest of the stars in Wilson's sample were either inactive, leading astronomers to wonder if these stars might not be in their own solar-like Maunder Minimum stage, or so chaotically active as to mask any regular cycle.

Upon closer examination, it turned out that these irregular stars were invariably young and highly active, while the stars displaying regular cycles were older, closer in age to our own sun's 4.5 billion years. "So it seems that stars are a lot like people," comments Duncan, who is today in charge of Wilson's original project. (As a graduate student, he was inspired to get involved in the field by one of Wilson's lectures.) "The younger the star, the more the activity. Younger stars are also far more erratic than older stars."

Since the sun is in every way a typical star, these findings gave astronomers an insight into the sun's early history. In its youth, the sun was probably far more active and its cycle far more chaotic than it is today. Now what puzzles astrophysicists is just how it "matured" to its current stage. They suspect it has to do with a slower rotation rate. Much as ice skaters slow down when they throw out their arms, the sun probably slowed down through a loss of angular momentum created by the outflow of particles in the solar wind.

By the time Wilson retired in 1977, the HK Project had become a hot property. "I guess in a sense I'm the guy who first climbed this Everest," says Wilson. "But since I did it they've now built a hotel up there and they are doing a good business."

Solar-stellar astronomy also got a boost from the discoveries made by a pair of satellites, both launched by the United States in 1978. One, the International Ultraviolet Explorer, sent back data showing that the chromospheres of stars in the solar neighborhood emitted in the ultraviolet; the other, the Einstein X-ray satellite, much to everyone's surprise, showed enormous X-ray emissions from the coronas, or outermost atmospheres, of these same stars. "Suddenly," says Duncan, "people realized that here was a wealth of information about what was going on in stars. Astronomers could begin talking about the density of high-energy material around stars and modeling their chromospheres and coronas the same way that solar astronomers try and model the sun's."

When Wilson retired, the HK Project fell into the hands of George Preston, director of the Mount Wilson and Las Campanas Observatories, and Arthur Vaughan, a stellar astronomer who considers himself "a mechanic with an interest in nature." Vaughan had heard about Wilson's work a few years previously, and had constructed an instrument to take the drudgery out of using the one-hundred-inch's spectrum scanner. What he built was the HK photometer, now installed on Mount Wilson's sixty-inch telescope. It measures with great precision the fluctuations in the two calcium wavelengths and compares them to the overall fluctuations in the spectrum, which result either from equipment instabilities or observation conditions. By subtracting the overall flux from the flux in the calcium readings stable readings could be assured.

With the new instrument, additional funding, and the participation of a few more astronomers, the HK project entered a new phase in the summer of 1980. The first problem they wanted to tackle involved a few puzzling variations that had appeared in Wilson's plots of stellar activity cycles. To solve it, they decided to take readings of the stellar emissions on a daily rather than monthly basis. Within months, they realized that the variations in the data resulted from the rotation of the stars.

Apparently, a large, magnetically-active region was causing the emission to jump every time the star rotated into view of the observing instrument. It was like measuring the rotation time of a distant lighthouse beacon by the appearance of its light. The rotation periods, which varied from a rapid 2.5 days in some stars to a lethargic 48 days in others, are a fundamental parameter in all theories attempting to account for the solar-magnetic cycle.

Shortly after this finding was made, Robert Noyes, an astrophysicist at the Harvard-Smithsonian Center for Astrophysics, along with colleagues there and at Mount Wilson, made what some say is the project's most fundamental discovery. They noticed that a star's rotation appeared to be linked to its activity; stars with regular cycles, like the sun, appear to rotate slowly, also like the sun. But a closer look indicated that among stars with the same rotation rate, some were much more active than others. To Noyes, this suggested that yet another factor, something other than rotation, was responsible for a star's activity. That factor has to do with just how fast a star radiates its energy.

Stars produce their energy through nuclear reactions at their core, and when a star is very hot it simply radiates its energy by bouncing it out atom by atom. But cooler stars, being more opaque, cannot radiate their energy fast enough and convection occurs near the surface. This process, explains Noyes, is quite similar to what happens in a bowl of bubbling oatmeal; the material on the bottom begins to heat up and expand, which makes it less dense than the material above it, until finally it rises and bubbles to the surface.

This convective activity is clearly visible on the sun through optical telescopes. Its surface is covered by thousands of individual granules, each about the size of the state of Texas, which are the tops of the convection cells. Astronomers believe that the outermost 30 percent of the sun is convective. Stars a little cooler than the sun are thought to have convective zones all the way through to their center.

So the best measure of a star's activity, Noyes concluded, takes into account both its rotation rate and the depth of its convection zone. This finding lends new support to long-standing theories that the twisting and kinking of the sun's magnetic fields by these rotational and convective motions might be sufficient to produce those mysterious sunspots.

"On some very cool dwarf stars, we think that half the star is covered with a spot," says Andrea Dupree of the Harvard-Smithsonian Center for Astrophysics. "This is just mindblowing to the pure theoretician. How do you have a magnetic field that literally comes out of half the side of a star? We are not even sure how to write down the equations for that kind of thing." But knowing that deep convection might be involved, as well as rotation rate, may help provide some answers.

Adding even more twists to our understanding of sunspots is that the sun rotates differentially, which means that it spins faster at the equator than at the poles. Could this differential rotation be found on other stars? Sallie Baliunas of the Center for Astrophysics thought that it could. But while the sun's differential rotation is easily observed by following the motion of sunspots through its eleven-year cycle, other stars are too distant for such direct observation. Once again the evidence had to come indirectly, from the variability of a star's calcium emissions.

"What we did is measure the change in period of rotation at different phases of the star's activity cycle," explains Baliunas. "Imagine that an active region of a star spins at a high latitude and marks out a period of fifteen days. The next season, if an active region appears at a lower latitude, one that is spinning faster, it marks out a shorter period, say twelve days. We are beginning to see these systematic changes, this progression of period, in about a dozen stars."

The precise monitoring of a star's calcium emission is about to unlock yet another stellar puzzle. What would happen, the HK team wondered, if you followed the activity of a single star over an entire night? Wilson had looked at the stars once a month and found their long cycles of activity. Vaughan had looked at the stars on a daily basis and found their rotational periods. What would a star's activity over the course of a single night tell you? The HK team thought it would tell them something about its interior.

Once again, astronomers turned to the sun as their Rosetta stone. "The sun's surface actually bobs up and down, like waves on an ocean, with a frequency of about five minutes," explains Baliunas. "This periodicity is the 'ringing' of the convective zone. So by knowing the frequency, we know how far the waves have travelled and how deep the convective zone really is. Now what we have been trying to do is measure this ringing on other stars. We look to see if the HK emission bobs up and down with some characteristic frequency."

Recent observations have led astronomers to believe that they now have their first detection of the oscillations from another star, ϵ Eridani, which is located about ten light-years away from the Earth. "We think we see the characteristic ringing in this star," says Baliunas. "The frequency is about ten minutes." Yet the depth of its convection zone remains unknown at the moment because this ten-minute frequency happens to be a combination of many different waves.

Baliunas explains: "The sun and stars have individual modes of vibrating. When you hear a bell you hear all different kinds of frequencies. So this ringing is a result of the waves that travel around the circumference of the star as well as those that travel longitudinally and radially. What we have to do is decompose this frequency by making more accurate measurements. And to do that, we really need an instrument that's ten times more accurate." Before developing a new instrument, however, the HK team will first try to modify their existing equipment.

Despite this limitation, the HK project's potential is far from being exhausted. When Duncan began running the day-to-day affairs of the project four years ago, the astronomers decided to expand the observing program to about a thousand stars. Among the new stars on the schedule since last year are the giants, those in the next stage in the process of stellar evolution for dwarf stars like the sun. Looking at giants is, in a sense, like looking at the future, though it will take another five billion years before our sun turns into one of these huge, bloated stars.

Duncan wanted to know what happens to dwarf stars when they become giants. How much do they slow down? What happens to their activity cycles? Do they continue? The results thus far show giants to have a wide range of activity, which leads him to believe that, given enough time, the team will find activity cycles in giants. But the data on the rotation of giants are in already; they show for the first time giants with rotation times as slow as a year. Chalk up another success for the HK project.

The ingenious astronomy behind the HK Project has gone a long way in shedding the sun and stars of many of their essential mysteries. But the insights from those key calcium emissions are but a preview of things to come. "By the 1990s," says astrophysicist Dupree confidently, "with the new instruments we are developing and the ability to observe from space, I expect we will be looking at the surfaces of stars with the same kind of detail that we now see on the sun."

HEART OF THE GALAXY

The next clear, late-summer night, cast your eyes skyward at the constellation Sagittarius in the southern portion of the sky. You are now looking toward the center of our galaxy, the Milky Way. Astronomers focusing on this very spot have produced the first detailed views of the galactic center. It shows a supernova remnant, a spiral-shaped region never before seen in our galaxy, and a point source believed to be the galaxy's actual nucleus. What's more, these images, when taken in conjunction with infrared and gamma ray observations, suggest that the nucleus of our galaxy may be a black hole.

For radio astronomers, it's all quite a coup. Never before have their colleagues been able to obtain a good view of the center of the Milky Way, as the galactic center has always been obscured to optical telescopes by the enormous cloud of interstellar dust that lies between the Earth and the center of the galaxy. But this dust, which all but blocks out the visual portion of the electromagnetic spectrum, has no effect on the radio waves that are emitted by the hot gases in the region and picked up by radio telescopes on Earth.

No longer is the center of our galaxy the quiet place astronomers have made it out to be in the past. Observations now show that it exhibits the kind of astrophysical pyrotechnics more normally associated with the active galaxies and quasars in the far regions of the cosmos. Galactic centers are dense regions where stars are born, die and then seem to fall together and collapse into compact, high-energy objects resembling the astrophysical models of black holes. A black hole is, by definition, invisible because its incredible gravitational force prevents even light from escaping its boundary.

So how can astronomers detect a black hole? By the unique radiation signature it leaves behind as it swallows up all the matter in its neighborhood. Matter falling toward a black hole at an angle forms a disk that rotates around it; as the matter spirals in and increases speed, it is heated to tremendous temperatures and gives off radiation.

If the nucleus of our galaxy is a black hole, it is certainly the biggest black hole in the galaxy. Yet it is quite small in comparison with the black holes that may reside in the centers of other galaxies. Their central engines may be millions of times more powerful than our own.

"If you were more than a few hundred light-years away from the black hole in the center of our galaxy you wouldn't even know it existed," says astronomer Robert Brown, of the National Radio Astronomy Observatory in Charlottesville, Virginia. "We, being 30,000 light-years away from the center and 20,000 light-years from the outer rim, are neither in any danger nor is it going to influence us in any way." But in cosmic terms, the black hole is right in our own back yard, and this proximity is a great advantage to astronomers hoping to unravel the complex nature of these exotic objects.

Astronomers are also intrigued by the other structures that lie near the center of the galaxy. A region of hot, ionized gas that appears as a green spiral in the radio images stretches ten light-years from one end to the other. Never before have astronomers seen this kind of gas in the form of a spiral in our galaxy. "It shows that the center of the galaxy is a very remarkable place," says Ron Ekers, director of the Very Large Array in New Mexico. The array's twenty-seven radio dishes are responsible for the remarkable new images of the galactic center. Studies by Brown of the movement of gases in this region suggests that the central object may be spewing out narrow jets of hot, gassy material in opposite directions as it rotates.

Astonomers also think they may have detected the outer envelopes of a supernova near the center of the galaxy. This remnant, which is typically generated when a star uses up its last remaining fuel and explodes, appears as a faint blue shell in radio images. Its location, however, puzzles astronomers.

"Why," asks Ekers, "is it so close and yet not right at the center of the galaxy? It just may be an accident that it appears as close as it does, but I doubt it." Perhaps, Ekers ventures when pressed for an explanation, galactic centers may normally be quiescent until nearby supernovas push enormous amounts of material in their black holes. With this kind of cosmic spark the galactic centers burst into activity.

The latest images of the Milky Way center reveal yet another unique astronomical structure, an arc more than 130 light-years long. The arc, which is formed of multiple parallel filaments, actually protrudes vertically from the plane of the galaxy. This large arc is linked to the core region by several shorter arcs. Their curvature suggests they were formed by particles trapped in some extremely strong magnetic fields.

Speculation as to what might lie at the center of the Milky Way began about two hundred years ago. At that time astronomers placed the Earth and the rest of the solar system near the center of the galaxy. That was the view of Sir William Herschel, the great astronomer in the court of King George III of England. Herschel, who boasted of seeing farther than any human before him, had counted the stars in the Milky Way and found an apparently equal number in all directions from Earth. His conclusion, reasonably enough, was that we were near the center of the galaxy.

Then about seventy years ago astronomers began to realize that we were actually located way out in the galaxy's suburbs, tens of thousands of light-years away from the center. It was astronomer Harlow Shapley who dared to propose that the center of the Milky Way lay in the direction of the constellation Sagittarius. He remained convinced, however, that the Milky Way was all there was to the Universe. Not until Edwin Hubble came along a few years later and applied the Doppler effect (the shift of red light coming from objects speeding toward or away from Earth) to measure distances on a cosmic scale was the Milky Way perceived as we perceive it today, as one of the thousands of millions of galaxies in the Universe.

Shapley had been correct about the direction of the center of the galaxy and Hubble correct about the distance, but only within the past few years have astronomers been able to determine whether the galactic center is a single, unusually bright source or a very dense cluster of stars. This determination came in part from the observations of Bruce Balick, of the University of Washington, and Robert Brown, who observed the radio waves emanating from the galactic center. While stationed at the Green Bank radio telescope in West Virginia back in 1974, Brown and Balick detected a very small source of radio emissions in that reigon. Brown and others have been measuring the fluctuations of that source ever since.

The source seems to vary in strength from year to year, from month to month, even from day to day. But never does it vary from minute to minute. Calculations based on these observations gave Brown and Balick a source that measured one light-day across, or no bigger than the diameter of the orbit of Jupiter. On a cosmic scale, that's small potatoes.

Then Ian Gatley, of the United Kingdom Infrared Telescope in Hawaii, measured the energy output of the galactic center. Using NASA's Kuiper Airborn Observatory (a modified C-41 that can carry an infrared telescope to very high altitudes) Gatley found that the luminosity of the galactic center is about ten million times the luminosity of the sun. Infrared maps of the galactic nucleus, which are based on heat energy emitted by dust particles irradiated by emissions from the nucleus, look very much like radio maps. It seems that the infrared-emitting dust and radio-wave-emitting gas must be complementary parts of the same structure.

What does that tell us? "Not much," says Brown, "just that where there is gas there is dust, and that the dust is hot and that something is heating it. The question is: What is heating it?" Is it a dense cluster of stars equal to ten million suns? Or is it a single object emitting the energy equivalent of ten million suns?

Gatley's observation confirmed the single-object theory in one quick stroke. "We all know that the closer you sit to the fire the hotter it gets," he says. "So a map of the distribution of the temperatures in the dust at the galactic source should allow us to see where the source or sources that radiate this power are located. The exciting result is that the temperature distribution is circularly symmetric and peaks in the center." It looks like a bull's eye with its brightest spot in the middle. And Gatley's hot spot happens to coincide with the point source in the radio image. There are no doubts now that the galactic center consists of a single powerful object.

Now that astronomers knew how big the galactic nucleus was and how much energy it emitted, figuring out what it was came quite easily. Astronomers simply asked themselves: What type of object has that kind of luminosity and is that small? Nothing but a black hole emits so much energy in such a small size. "The conclusion has to be that the center of the galaxy is either a black hole or some object closely related to it," says Brown. "At this point, the answer is more a matter of semantics than physics."

The case for the black hole becomes particularly compelling when you consider the evidence, gathered by balloon and satellite observations, of gamma rays that seem to be emanating from the core of the galaxy. "This thing is the brightest gamma-ray object in the galaxy," says Bell Laboratories astrophysicist Marvin Leventhal. "If you were to look up at the galaxy with gamma-ray sensitive eyes, you would see the galactic center and not much else." These data indicate that the galactic center is a profuse producer of positrons (antielectrons) and a powerful source of gamma rays that fluctuates in a time span of about six months. The only kind of object that we know about in the universe that could emit so many gamma rays, make positrons in such great numbers and fluctuate in such a short time frame is a black hole swallowing large amounts of matter.

These observations also hint at a possible future for the Milky Way. The evidence from gamma rays suggests that the object at the galactic core contains between one hundred and one million solar masses. Some scientists have speculated that an object of such great mass could have unusual properties. According to a theory proposed by Leonid Ozernoi, a Russian astrophysicist, one hundred solar masses is the threshold point of black hole development. Ozernoi believes that a black hole that begins at less than one hundred solar masses will consume only its immediate surroundings. But if the black hole starts out at more than one hundred solar masses, it will continue to devour everything nearby until it develops to quasar size. If the center of the galaxy is a black hole of this size, and if Ozernoi is correct, then the Milky Way might someday become a quasar.

A bright future indeed!

FOUNTAINS OF SPACE

Every morning a pair of dust-covered buses heads west from the small mining town of Socorro, New Mexico, carrying their loads of astronomers, engineers, computer operators, technicians and support personnel on the hour-long journey into the desert. Their destination is the largest and most powerful radio telescope in the world, the Very Large Array or, as it is affectionately called by the astronomers who use it to study the farthest reaches of the cosmos, the VLA.

Located amid rolling tumbleweed, rattlesnakes and cattle feeding on the sparse vegetation of the Plains of San Augustin, the massive white bowls of the VLA point skyward, recording the hissing and the moaning of all the strange beasts in the cosmic zoo. When all twenty-seven dish antennas that make up the VLA are coordinated and focused on the same point in the heavens, they become a single instrument with the power of a conventional radio telescope with a dish as large in diameter as the Capital Beltway that surrounds Washington, D.C., twenty-one miles.

The VLA's dish antennas are spread out on this ancient lake bed along three arms of an immense Y-shaped railroad track. Each dish measures 82 feet in diameter and weighs 212 tons. During the day, if you are patient, you may notice the slow sluing motion of the dishes as they swivel with ballet-like precision in their search for astronomical wonders in the depths of space. The VLA is not hampered by cloud cover or daylight and can operate twenty-four hours a day for unlike its optical brethren it gathers no light. Instead, like all radio telescopes, it observes a different portion of the electromagnetic spectrum, radio waves. The sun, moon and most of the planets emit radio signals, as do pulsars, quasars, supernovas and the vast clouds of gas and organic molecules that coalesce into stars in space.

Once an astronomer decides which source of radio waves he or she wants to observe and makes certain decisions regarding wavelength, bandwidth and calibration, a series of computers (called by such names as Boss, Monty and Eunice) actually aim the telescope and store, measure and analyze the data that the great dishes collect. The final product, in many cases, is a picture or, as radio astronomers call it, a map of radio sources that appear as sharp as objects in photographs taken by the world's most powerful optical telescopes.

With a sky full of radio sources, not all of which can be seen with an optical telescope, there is much to keep the VLA astronomers busy. But of all the strange beasts that inhabit the cosmic zoo, none are more impressive than the enormous radio sources associated with some quasars and elliptical galaxies. Astronomers call these sources radio quasars and radio galaxies. When they can be seen through an optical telescope, the "parent" galaxies from which radio galaxies emanate appear to be nothing out of the ordinary. Through a large radio telescope, however, these radio galaxies appear to consist of a central core galaxy and a huge symmetrical pair of lobes that seem to have exploded out of the core. Some of these radio galaxies appear to span as much as one hundred million trillion miles, dwarfing the optical, or parent galaxies from which they emanate.

"They are the largest, the furthest, the most powerful, and to some of us, the most fascinating objects in the Universe," says George Miley, the world-renowned radio astronomer from the Netherlands. "They are also objects of considerable beauty."

The first radio galaxies were observed more than a quarter of a century ago when astronomers discovered an incredibly powerful radio source called Cygnus A. With its dumbbell-like shape, Cygnus A was unlike any cosmic beast ever seen. The radio picture showed a large region of emission beyond each edge of the parent galaxy with which it was associated. Bright regions, or hot spots, glowed in each of these two radio lobes, as the regions of extended emission are called. And by the 1960s, improved instrumentation showed that a very small radio source was also embedded inside the core of Cygnus A. Once it was established that this odd structure, two lobes and a core, was common among radio galaxies, astronomers began to realize that their optical portraits of galaxies had been telling only part of the story.

Radio galaxies present astronomers with a twofold scientific mystery. First and foremost, they wondered how these sources could generate such enormous amounts of energy. They hoped to find a clue to this mystery by first finding out how this energy was being transferred from the core of the galaxy to the outer lobes, which are located hundreds of thousands of light years away.

During the 1960s, scientists envisioned a variety of simple models to explain these features. Two opposing models drew the most attention. According to one, the core of the galaxy was ejecting blobs of matter like Puffed Wheat shot from a cannon. But the tremendous loss of energy in such an expanding cloud could not supply the energy clearly present in the hot spots. Besides, astronomers wondered, how do you suddenly blow out 10 percent of the galaxy's energy without blowing it apart? That was just asking too much.

The other approach, proposed by Martin Rees, of Cambridge in England and director of the Institute of Astronomy, suggested that an invisible energy pipeline ran from the core to the lobes carrying a continuous supply of energy. He called these hypothetical energy channels "beams" or "jets." The concept seemed attractive to chalk-and-blackboard astronomers, and the search for the "radio jets" was on.

Astonomers first began looking for these jets in high-luminosity radio sources such as Cygnus A, because it was the enormous energy needs of these lobes that had led to the jet theory in the first place. But that's not where radio jets were found. Instead, they were discovered quite by accident in a lower luminosity source, 3C219, by Cambridge radio astronomer Brian Turland.

"The striking feature," Turland wrote in the monthly notices of the Royal Astronomical Society, "is the presence of a central radio component which, unlike most others, consists of a compact source centered on the galaxy and a 'jet' pointing along the axis of the source as defined by the high brightness regions of the outer components. This is the first time that such a jet has been found to be associated with a classical double radio source."

Once this cosmic missing link had been found, astronomers

noticed that some of their older radio maps had shown hints of such jet-like structures. Ironically, a jet-like feature had already been seen with an optical telescope in the elliptical galaxy M87 as early as 1910. Only at that time radio sources were not even known to exist, and the feature was passed over as an oddity.

Turland's observation and those that followed provided circumstantial evidence in favor of a jet-type model, and scientists began to feel they might be able to understand the mystery of how all that energy was transported hundreds of thousands of light-years out to the lobes. For scientists, the discovery of these jets presented a satisfying picture of an observation answering a theoretical need. "I think the most interesting thing about this discovery was that jets had been predicted some five years before they were found," says astronomer Ron Ekers, who was at Cambridge while the theoretical work was being done and is now the VLA site director. "That happens rather infrequently in science."

Radio jets were suddenly a hot topic; they were the talk of the scientific community. To astronomers the topic was sexy, and before long the handful or so who took up the study of radio jets became known, not surprisingly, as the jet set. They included such people as Ed Fomalont, Rick Perley, George Miley, Wil van Breugel, Tony Willis and Alan Bridle.

Much of what we know about radio jets today comes from the jet set's use of the VLA, which became operational in 1976 but was completed only in 1980. "It suddenly showed that radio jets were very common and occur in lots of sources," says Ekers. Nobody had appreciated how dominant they would be and how interesting their shapes were until astronomers began aiming the VLA dishes at them in 1977. At that time, with just nine of the twenty-seven antennas operational, the VLA already possessed more collecting power than any other instrument of its kind. The array's high resolution, its ability to distinguish faint features in the midst of bright emission, was perfectly adapted to studying these unusual sources.

Radio jets appear to be made up of a hot gas, or plasma (clouds of energetic electrons moving in magnetic fields at close to the speed of light). Flowing along with this plasma is a cooler gas that does not radiate. Even when taken together, however, the matter densities are low, so that if you could somehow sample the environment, you would find only a few electrons per cubic centimeter.

Jets become visible near the core of a radio galaxy, after a "gap" of a few thousand parsecs. (A parsec equals 19.2 trillion miles, or 206,451 times the distance between the Earth and the Sun.) Then they open up into tube-like structures as they extend to the outer lobes. Their lengths vary from just a few parsecs to more than a million. The hot spots in the lobes seem to represent the ends of the jet beams.

In the more feeble radio sources the jets expand more rapidly and produce larger, more amorphous hot spots, hinting at a relatively slow velocity of materials in these jets. Their visibility to radio telescopes also attests to an inefficiency, indicating that the jets have lost most of their energy on the way to the lobes. Scientists use this efficiency argument to explain why the jets in powerful radio sources and quasars are so often invisible. They reason that the stronger the source, the more efficient the jet. This means that it radiates less energy on the way to the lobe and produces very small, but more intense, hot spots.

Radio jets vary considerably in shape. Some are straight as a laser beam, while others bend or twist like a corkscrew, as if they had been ejected from a rotating source. Many seem to wiggle, perhaps because of the motion of the source through the intergalactic medium. But just how the jets remain confined over such long distances and why they remain internally unperturbed when bent is still a source of wonder for the astronomer.

Variations in the jets (shape, brightness and width) provide scientists with a kind of evolutionary record of the motion of these extragalactic sources through the environment. "Headtail" sources, which are bent into the shape of a horseshoe and whose discovery actually preceded that of the jets themselves, are startling examples of such environmental effects. Observations on the VLA have made clear that these tails form when a normal dumbbell radio source is swept back by the motion of its parent galaxy through a dense, intergalactic medium.

To astronomers like Rick Perley, these distorted sources are worth their weight in gold. "These are fun objects," he says, "because you get a chance to do physics on them." But in some astronomy circles, use of jets to probe the source's environment has been known, somewhat derogatorily, as "weather forecasting." Looking at the "weather" around a source is not terribly interesting to those astronomers whose goal it is to see the beast naked. They want to see radio sources as they really are, to see those sources that are too powerful to be affected by the environment. The not-so-obscure objects of their desire are high-luminosity sources such as quasars, bodies that appear to be the size of stars but emitting the energy of a billion stars. Quasars may be galaxies in which the core has become very active, pouring out huge amounts of energy. Quasars are a noticeable fraction of the age of the Universe and the most distant objects from the Earth.

The symmetries of radio jets may provide certain clues to the nature of these most powerful energy sources in the Universe. While feeble radio galaxies generally have jets emerging from opposite sides of the core, jets shoot out from powerful radio galaxies more rarely, and then usually only from one side. Why the jets go to one side when the lobes they are feeding are on both sides is one of the major unresolved problems in the field.

The puzzle has several possible explanations. The first is that the nuclear engine in the core of the galaxy flip-flops, supplying energy first to one lobe, then to the other. Another explanation is that the properties of the environment differ on each side, allowing jets to be seen on one side but not the other. Yet a third explanation calls for a "Doppler favoritism" in which the jet moving toward the observer at close to the speed of light becomes brighter, while the one moving away becomes so dim as to be invisible.

How to explain the tremendous energy that pours from these high-power sources may be the ultimate problem in radio astronomy today. What is the nature of the engine that drives the radio jets? To answer that question, theorists have pulled out of the hat astronomy's favorite rabbit, the black hole. They believe that inside the tiny cores, which can be one-millionth the size of the overall source, are spinning black holes, each equal in mass to millions of suns. Gases spiraling into a black hole probably form a disk from which energy is squirted out along its rotation axis, producing the jets.

One of the strongest pieces of evidence that black holes might be the engines that power these extragalactic sources comes from a denizen of our own Milky Way. The object, known as SS433, may be an effective Rosetta Stone for understanding the physics of those far-out jet sources. SS433 intrigues astronomers because the changes in this source take place on a time scale of hours and months rather than the millions of years that extragalactic sources require.

SS433 created a sensation in 1979 when two English astronomers working in Australia found unusually strong radio and X-ray emissions coming from this bizarre source. What tantalized scientists was that the object appeared to be simultaneously approaching and receding at tremendous speeds. They likened it to a giant lawn sprinkler, spewing out tongues of gas.

"I initially didn't want to look at SS433 at all, because it was clear that every glory-grabber in the world was jumping on this bandwagon," says Bob Hjellming, a specialist in stellar radio emission at the VLA. But he soon realized that here was one of the most explicit cases available in which he could study changes in the characteristics of the jets. So Hjellming jumped into the fray with the assistance of Ken Johnson, of the Hulburt Center for Space Research in Washington, D.C. Together, using the VLA, they produced the first series of good high-resolution maps of SS433.

Hjellming calls SS433 "the little engine that could" because it actually does on a small scale everything the central object in extragalactic radio sources had always been suspected of doing. "What makes SS433 really exciting is the level of detail we are getting about what is happening," he says. "And in this case more than any other we are nearly certain just what the root cause is of the phenomenon we are seeing." Hjellming and colleagues think that SS433 is a neutron star, a star that has collapsed into an extremely dense mass, or perhaps a black hole that has collapsed even farther in a binary system with a normal star. The normal star is dumping mass on this compact object, whose rotational energy ejects a radio-emitting flow of plasma in the form of a corkscrew.

In the future, the VLA is expected to yield many more answers to the problems posed by these incredible energy sources—and many new surprises as well. "Something which strikes me as being particularly true of radio astronomy is the amount of accidental discovery that has always occurred," says Ekers. "There are a huge number of examples. Pulsars, quasars and the three-degree background radiation that permeates the Universe and seems to be an 'echo' of the Big Bang were all major discoveries made in this way. No theoretical prediction led to their discoveries. They were entirely new phenomena that opened up whole new fields. And this has been largely a result of instrumentation, which has always dominated progress in radio astronomy. A good instrument like the VLA may be more important than the people who use it."

Once a discovery is made, however, it isn't long before the field of study it spawns is taken for granted. Such a fate has already befallen radio jets. The glamour of those "fountains of radio stuff," as MIT astrophysicist Philip Morrison calls radio jets, has given way to the enormous amount of hard work that remains before scientists understand radio galaxies.

"Radio jets have been worked to death," says Tim Cornwell, an assistant scientist at the VLA. With a burst of laughter, he adds: "Now we know that we don't understand them."

FRONTIERS

INVESTIGATORS OF THE TWILIGHT ZONE

The scent of honeysuckle drifted through the hot and humid air. It was summer, and amid the classical pavilions and sweeping lawns of the University of Virginia, a scientific conference was taking place. But this was no ordinary scientific conference. The dean of an Ivy League school of engineering and applied science was talking about his experiments with psychic phenomena. One of the most respected astrophysicists in the country was discussing the problems facing UFO research. And a zoologist was holding an audience of fellow scientists spellbound with the details of his search for a prehistoric dinosaur deep in the jungles of Africa.

The occasion was the second annual meeting of the Society for Scientific Exploration (SSE). The eminent attendees, ranging from astronomers to zoologists, are all affiliated with universities or research institutions, yet their interests are as unorthodox as their credentials are solid. They came to share their knowledge and whet their curiosity about mysteries long of interest to the general public but which science in its noble search has tended to ignore. As one said, "They came here not for professional reasons, but for intellectual stimulation." UFOs, psychokinesis, astrology, all are fair game for these intrepid investigators of the Twilight Zone.

Peter Sturrock, a professor of space science and astrophysics at Stanford, is the society's president and founder. "If scientists are going to accept the task of trying to find responsible answers to anomalous phenomena," he explained, "it is essential that these claims be subjected to the normal processes of science and scholarship, including open debate, publication and criticism. That's what this society hopes to provide—a forum through which research on these questions may be presented to the community of scientists and scholars."

Debate was lively at the conference. One scientist presented a thorough analysis of what has been called the New Zealand UFO case. Discussing a 16-mm film of the purported UFO, he said the strange series of lights has no conventional explanation. But to another scientist, they looked like navigation lights. "If that's not the aircraft's beacon reflected off the propeller, I'll eat my hat," he said.

Each scientist appeared interested in one anomaly and tended to dismiss the rest. Said one historian: "I don't care about Bigfoot, ESP, and all of that. I'm only interested in UFOs." But while the scientists weren't all there for the same reason, they all risked the ridicule of their colleagues for taking such issues seriously. Yet, in a way, anomalies suit the spirit and challenges of scientific orthodoxy. One of the tasks of science has always been to explain the things that go bump in the night; to banish dragons and ghosts (or prove their existence) by bringing them under the clear light of scientific scrutiny.

The first topic to be scrutinized at the conference was Dr. Ian Stevenson's evidence on American children who claim to remember previous lives. Stevenson, who is a Carlson Professor of Psychiatry at the University of Virginia Medical Center, has travelled around the world in search of cases of alleged reincarnation. His talk took note of both the differences and the similarities between ninety-five American cases and the 235 cases he had collected from the Indian subcontinent.

Stevenson discovered that both the American and Indian children first recalled details of what appeared to be a previous life at about three years of age. Many children in both groups claimed to remember that their previous lives had ended in violent deaths, and almost half the children had developed phobias linked with the mode of that death.

But American children spontaneously stopped speaking of their experience at about the age of five, Stevenson noted, more than a year before the Indian children. He thinks this may be due to either inattention or suppression by elders. "The thought that the child might be in some ways deviant is terribly troubling to most American parents," he said. "There is a great concern that the child may be abnormal, which as you all know is a more serious crime than murder in the United States." For this reason Stevenson believes that American cases are seriously underreported.

Impressive as it had at first seemed, Stevenson's case for reincarnation began to unravel when he noted that American children rarely gave enough specific details of their experience to be able to identify the person whom they claimed to remember being. "In the cases where American children do give specifying details and we have verified the statements," said Stevenson, "these nearly always refer to someone in the child's own family."

This comment led one physicist to express privately grave doubts about the whole subject of reincarnation. "It's so easy for children to have access to information about previous members of their family," he said. "How can you be sure they didn't pick up the details from a conversation or a family photo album? Besides, if you have children, you know how prone children are to fantasies of all types."

In the discussion afterwards, one scientist objected to Stevenson's data on the basis that population estimates show that there were just not enough bodies available in the past for all the souls present today. Another scientist, admitting that the subject was far from his "normal habitat," wondered if fingerprint matches had ever been attempted. Stevenson replied that such data was not available.

SSE president Sturrock, who founded the Institute for Plasma Research at Stanford and who has been chairman of a National Academy of Science study panel on solar physics, is himself primarily interested in UFOs. But he emphasized the importance of a kind of holistic approach to the study of all anomalies. "Each of us has a great deal to learn from people in other fields," he said. In fact, Sturrock's presentation of the critical issues facing UFOlogy today are quite similar to the problems facing all areas of anomaly research, the basic issue being how to deal with the problem of nonreplicable events.

"Any scientific development goes through a gray stage between ignorance and understanding," said Sturrock. "I think the gray areas in science are the most interesting. The goal of scientific inference is to deal with uncertain knowledge, to deal with uncertain consequences and hypotheses. You don't try to establish the truth all at once, you simply try to see whether this block of imperfect data makes this hypothesis more or less uncertain. That's one way to make progress in the field anomalies."

Sturrock also decried a certain lack of courage among researchers of anomalies. "It is often mentioned in regard to anomalous phenomena that if you are going to be scientific you should not theorize," he said. "I don't subscribe to that view. I feel there is a great benefit to proposing hypotheses and theories as rapidly as possible. It's not necessary that any one of the theories be correct because they help organize and analyze data and provide a great stimulus for further research. Astronomers are not bashful about rushing into print with conjectures when new discoveries are made, and that's the way it should be."

A number of scientists were impressed by Michael Persinger's hypothesis that tectonic strain is the primary source of UFO-related luminosities or luminous displays. A neuroscientist at Laurentian University in Ontario, Canada, Persinger has found that UFO reports increase in number before earthquake activity. "As tectonic strain accumulates you get luminous displays," he explained, "and if the strain continues to increase you get earthquakes."

Persinger added that "the lights themselves may be a plasma-like condition surrounded by very intense magnetic fields," and that a close encounter with such a luminous display could produce a number of serious neurological effects such as hallucinations, paralysis or amnesia.

One scientist commented afterwards that Persinger's use of the word UFO might be misleading because his theory did not seem to explain all types of UFO reports. He suggested that Persinger might be better off using the term UAL, meaning unidentified aerial luminosities. Persinger agreed that his theory accommodates only certain types of UFO reports, but thought that United Air Lines might object to the use of the letters UAL in this way.

Dr. Bruce Greyson, a psychiatrist at the University of Michigan Medical Center in Ann Arbor, talked about another anomaly with a three-letter abbreviation. When speaking of his study of anomalous experiences following suicide attempts, Greyson was, of course, referring to near-death experiences, commonly known as NDEs. These are profound, often pleasurable, subjective experiences that some people report when they come close to dying.

Greyson set out to discover whether, as some people suspect, NDEs are a kind of psychopathology. "Many people assume that the NDE is a psychological defense against the threat of death," said Greyson, "or that it's some organic brain disfunction caused by coming close to death and being short of oxygen." But in analyzing the reports of sixty-one consecutive admissions for suicide attempts on a number of medical and psychological variables, Greyson found no evidence to suggest that NDEs represent a psychopathological state.

Asked afterwards if NDEs might not be perceived as a reward and might not therefore lead to repeated suicide attempts, Greyson replied: "We were worried about that, but, in fact, found just the opposite effect. Having an NDE makes people much less likely to repeat the suicide attempt. In talking to attemptors what they seem to say is that although the NDE does make death seem less frightening and more attractive, it also makes life more meaningful and purposeful."

Life may be meaningful for those experiencing NDEs, but for physicists things may look a little depressing, according to University of Oklahoma physicist Richard Fowler, who spoke about the decline in the growth of ideas in the field of physics. Fowler came to this conclusion after having first deduced population estimates for various periods of history, formulated a list of the great ideas in physics, and finally entered the figures in a formula he had devised, in which the accumulation of ideas grows exponentially with the number of man years lived. The result was somewhat surprising.

"It seems that since 1920 we have begun to fall deficient in ideas," Fowler stated. "We are short about a hundred ideas in physics. It looks vaguely as if physics is converging. Some say there is only one more neutrino to be found. Maybe physics is coming to an end." Commented one scientist in good humor: "I can think of an alternate explanation. Maybe the human mind is coming to an end."

The anomalies discussed at the conference have been thorns

in the side of science. They won't go away, and yet they have been notoriously difficult for science to handle. And, as James Trefil, professor of physics at the University of Virginia, points out, "It's important to know what the rules of the game are when dealing with the gray areas of science." Trefil has formulated three such rules.

Rule one is that a claim based on a single event will be rejected in science if an alternate explanation exists at probability levels on the order of one in a billion or one in a trillion. "To give you an idea of what that probability is," he explained, "if you had a die that came out successfully one time in a trillion, and you rolled it once a second, you would be rolling it for an appreciable fraction of the lifetime of the universe before it came up right."

His second rule states that if there is no acceptable alternative explanation, an event remains in limbo if it leads to severe theoretical difficulties. "You shouldn't feel miffed if your event gets put in limbo," Trefil told his fellow scientists. "There is no disgrace in being in limbo, and until theoretical problems are resolved you may get stuck there."

Trefil's third rule says that a claim based on many events will be rejected if each event taken individually is statistically insignificant. "That's one of the problems with UFO research," said Trefil. "There may be lots of evidence, but each event, taken by itself, is shaky."

One scientist who seems to have the rules of the game well in hand is Robert Jahn, the dean of the school of engineering and applied science at Princeton University. While the bulk of Jahn's research activities at Princeton involves fluid mechanics, ionized gases, electric propulsion and other topics in the aerospace sciences, during the past few years he has brought his knowledge of engineering to bear on a series of experiments in controlled, low-level psychokinesis (PK), the alleged ability of human consciousness to affect the behavior of physical systems in a verifiable way.

What distinguishes Jahn's experiments from most other psychic research is his use of high technology apparatus to produce technically impeccable experiments with extremely large data bases. He and his associate, Brenda Dunn, have run tens of thousands of trials in which subjects have significantly shifted the mean distribution of two devices, one that randomly generates electronic signals, the other a random mechanical cascade.

The latter experiment utilizes a pinball device that allows 9,000 three-quarter-inch marbles to circulate around 350 nylon pegs and distribute themselves into nineteen collecting bins at the bottom. Some subjects have successfully influenced the distribution of the marbles to either the left or the right of the mean baseline distribution. "In both machines, we see a very marginal shift of means from the chance expectation and from the empirical baseline," said Jahn. "The significance of that marginal shift becomes evident only after we accumulate very large data bases."

The conclusion Jahn draws from these experiments is both cautious and startling. "The two machines are very different but the results are similar," he says, "and it may be that the process of interaction operates at the level of the output information rather than at the level of the random physical process itself. Therefore, what we may be dealing with in PK is more a transfer of information than a transfer of energy."

Another type of contemporary psychic research covered at the SSE meeting was remote viewing. In a typical remote viewing experiment the subject is asked to describe a remote, unknown location where an outbound "agent" has been sent and with whom there is no normal communication during the course of the experiment. Afterwards, independent judges attempt to match the subject's descriptions with photographs of the actual target sites. Among those speaking on the subject was Hal Puthoff, a physicist at the radiophysics laboratory at SRI International in Menlo Park, California.

"It's actually easier for people to describe a whole scene than it is for them to guess numbers or symbols on cards," said Puthoff, who after a decade of such experiments devised the "two-thirds, two-thirds, one-half" rule of remote viewing. "What this means," said Puthoff, "is that if you grab a group of selected people, roughly two out of three will generate significant results. When you look at anyone of those people, basically two-thirds of their data will be good or accurate. And if you look at the data overall in terms of what gets matched in various blind-matching procedures, roughly one-half of the sites will get blind-matched to their corresponding targets."

After the initial series of experiments, Puthoff became convinced of the reality of the phenomenon and took a closer look at both the subjects and their data. His attempt to profile the distinguishing characteristics of the good remote viewer got nowhere. After subjecting his subjects to a variety of physiological, psychological and neuropsychological tests, he found that good remote viewers did not differ significantly from the normal population. But an analysis of the remote viewing data itself gave some insight into the process. "Good data tends to come first at the feeling level," said Puthoff, "and only then develops into a visual image. If, for instance, a subject starts out saying that he got a flash of Manhattan Island, you can be almost sure that's noise."

At the end of his presentation Puthoff tried to counter many of the criticisms that have been aimed at his work, but at least one scientist remained unconvinced. "Puthoff is getting government funding," said the dubious scientist, "and that makes me wonder if all his material might not be some sort of government disinformation to mislead the Russians into wasting time and money on this apparent breakthrough."

Not all the presentations were quite so controversial. A dozen years ago MIT atmospheric scientist Ralph Markson was invited to speak on the subject of sun-weather relationships for a scientific program's controversial slot in Madrid. Markson's hypothesis that solar variability modifies weather through an atmospheric electrical process tends to raise eyebrows among scientists because the only recognized solar effect on weather at the moment depends on change in solar heating. But when he delivered a paper on the same subject amid SSE's highly controversial program of speakers, the subject seemed relatively tame.

"What first attracted me to the idea of atmospheric electricity thirty years ago," said Markson, "was the knowledge that the Earth's electric field changes simultaneously all over the world. Now we've found that the variability of the solar wind is highly correlated with the intensity of the Earth's electric field. The missing link in the problem is how do changes in the electric field affect the weather? I think the answer lies in cloud physics. That's the only viable way of influencing weather on a short time scale."

Markson believes that solar variability modulates the

earth's electric field by controlling ionizing radiation through global thunderstorm activity. Asked by Sturrock what the chances were that this effect was real, Markson replied: "Well, we can fool ourselves, but I wouldn't be spending my life working on this if I didn't think it was real." If Markson turns out to be correct, his research may one day result in marked improvements in both short-term and long-term weather forecasting.

Science is sometimes more than a matter of abstract concepts and numbers. As Roy Mackal's presentation made quite clear, it can be pure adventure as well. In his survey of cryptozoology, the zoologist from the University of Chicago gave an account of his hazardous search for the existence of a large, mysterious water beast known to the natives of the Central African swamp-forests as the Mokele-Mbembe. The animal is said to be brownish-gray in color and hairless, with a long, flexible neck and a thick tail.

For the last two hundred years the natives have reported not only seeing but killing several of the animals, which Mackal believes might be Mesozoic sauropods, a type of dinosaur that includes the seventy-foot brontosaurus. Since 1981 Mackal has headed two expeditions into the Likouala swamps of the People's Republic of the Congo, battling parasites, cholera and malaria, as well as a variety of poisonous snakes, looking for the animal that "makes footprints that require a body like that of a hippopotamus or an elephant, but with claws."

Mackal gave more details of his agonizing trek than of the mystery animal itself because he never managed to find the creature. He talked mostly of the heat, the task of obtaining permits from all the appropriate ministries, the meals of monkey meat captured by the pygmies, the pythons dropping from overhanging branches into their dugout canoes, and the need for Clorox in their drinking water. Mackal and his team of scientists also did traditional science along the way, mapping the area, collecting plants, photographing animals, and excavating artifacts from an archaeology site uncovered at Impfondo.

Other than bringing back some examples of what is said to be the mystery animal's staple food, the "molombo" fruit, Mackal also managed to collect some new anecdotal evidence of the elusive creature's existence. "We received information from over thirty individuals," he said. "That's what impressed me. They had different ethnic, religious, cultural and geographic backgrounds and yet the details of their description were identical. If this animal were a cultural or religious construction, I would expect it to be related to one tribe but not another."

The role and importance of skepticism in anomaly research was the topic of Marcello Truzzi's polemical presentation. "Science must be cautious yet remain open," said Truzzi, who is the head of the department of sociology at Eastern Michigan University in Ypsilanti. He began by pointing out the difference between disbelief, which is believing that something is not true, and nonbelief, which is a state of suspended judgment. "By definition, the skeptic should be a nonbeliever," said Truzzi, "neither believing something to be true nor believing it to be false. We must remember that the role of science is to explain, not to explain away, phenomena. Skepticism should be constructive, rather than purely destructive, which tends to block inquiry."

Truzzi gave a kind of pep talk to his audience of "endoheretics," a term used by Isaac Asimov to denote those within the professional world of science who hold perspectives deviant from those of their colleagues. "Those who complain about the unscientific status of psychic counselors," he said, taking a crack at the critics, "should also be willing to examine the scientific status of orthodox psychotherapy and make truly scientific comparisons.

"Those who sneer at holy prophets in our midst might also do well to look at the prognosticators in economics and sociology who hold official positions as scientific forecasters," he continued. "Those who concern themselves about newspaper horoscopes and their influence might do well to look at what the real so-called healthy professions are doing. The scientist who claims to be a true skeptic, a zetetic, should be willing to empirically investigate the claims of the American Medical Association as well as those of the faith healers."

The scientists who attended the meeting placed themselves in a somewhat precarious position—though that position is also one which holds great potential for new discoveries. Said Princeton's Robert Jahn: "My friend Edgar Mitchell, the astronaut, is very fond of saying that the fact that he had walked on the moon got him access to many offices and many persons—

once. I think that those of us who approach anomalies from within an established discipline have the same burden. We have access to the ears of our colleagues—once. But from that point on, depending on the credibility of the case and the objectivity of the audience, we may be regarded as a prophet, an annoyance, or, on the other extreme, a traitor."

The very need for an organization such as the Society for Scientific Exploration led MIT's Ralph Markson to bemoan the lack of curiosity among scientists and wonder if the scramble for funding had not turned science into a mere rat race. "What has happened to science?" he asked. "Why aren't there more scientists here? Anomalies are what science is all about."

SASQUATCH!

Professor Grover Krantz leans back in his chair and places his left foot on the seminar table where his five students are seated. This is not rudeness on the part of the bearded, fifty-three year-old anthropologist, but a demonstration of a problem in contemporary physical anthropology. Next to his left shoe, which measures twelve inches, he props up a plaster cast of an enormous footprint.

"This is a seventeen-inch-long Sasquatch track," says Krantz. "It's excessively wide and hopelessly out of the size range of a human foot. The absolute maximum size for a human foot is fifteen inches. I didn't put much likelihood into this creature being real until the spring of 1970 when I was able to get a hold of these casts."

The topic of discussion for this evening's graduate anthropology class at Washington State University in Pullman, Washington is Bigfoot, or Sasquatch as century-old Indian legends call the large hairy creature that supposedly stalks the Pacific Northwest. Though the university is highly regarded for its agriculture department, its wood-products research and its veterinary school, it is perhaps best known for the volume of alcohol its students consume and for its controversial professor of physical anthropology, Grover Krantz, who has been unabashedly pursuing the elusive Bigfoot for the past fifteen years.

Krantz is describing a creature which is considerably taller and heavier than his own 210-pound, 6-foot-3-inch frame. "What people usually report," he says, "is something seven to eight feet tall with an extremely heavy build—about 800 pounds—and covered with a fairly dense coat of brown or black hair two to four inches long. Its face has less hair or is naked; it looks somewhat like a gorilla's face, but much longer. Its shoulders are large and high, so that the mouth and chin are below shoulder level, which is a very ape-like characteristic. But it walks on two legs in a human manner, with the walking hinge, the hip joint, about mid-height. Bears have the walking hinge very much lower."

Reports of a large hairy primate living wild in North America and other parts of the world have persisted for over a century. In the Florida Everglades, it is known as the Skunk Ape because of its overwhelming stench. Sightings have also been reported in New England and the Great Lakes states. In China, where it is known as Wild Man, and in the Himalayas, where it is called Yeti, the creature is said to be somewhat smaller than Bigfoot.

"The most economical hypothesis is that all the reports involve the same species, with sub-species differences," says Krantz, adjusting his wire-rimmed glasses. "But I draw a distinction between what is going on in the Pacific Northwest and what is happening in other parts of the world. Here, I'm at it firsthand. I've talked to the people who have seen it, and I've seen the footprints."

Krantz's colleagues, less familiar with his work, are more skeptical. One primatologist says Krantz is working in an area "where angels fear to tread." Physical anthropologist Jack Kelso, of the University of Colorado, says: "I'm just not familiar with the evidence. He may be right, but I must say I'm a long way off from believing it myself."

Nevertheless, Krantz estimates that there are now about one thousand eyewitness reports of the creature. The actual number of sightings may be ten times that many, since most eyewitnesses tell very few people about what they saw. "Of the thirty-six eyewitnesses I've interviewed myself," he says, "I think that about half were either lying to me, were fooled by something else, saw something out of a whiskey bottle, or gave me information too poor to evaluate. With the other half, I couldn't find anything wrong."

Unlike the wild-eyed amateurs who dominate the Sasquatch

scene, Krantz is a rational and methodical scientist who is well aware of the limitations of eyewitness testimony. "If science accepted every creature on the testimony of ten or so sightings," he says, "then we would have a zoological inventory that included unicorns, goblins, griffins, fairies, and moth-men. But on the other hand, if even just one Sasquatch story is true, then the animal is real and the species is there."

And what if Sasquatch is real? "It would mean that science has completely missed one of the biggest and potentially most important mammalian species on earth," says Krantz. "Finding such a creature should also settle the question about upright posture having anything to do with intelligence and speech. But perhaps the most critical effect of such a find would be on an emotional level. If this is what I think it is, it's the closest living relative of human beings, closer than the great apes. That would make it the biological discovery of the century."

Krantz suspects that the Sasquatch is a living representative of *Gigantopithecus,* a giant primate known from the fossils of its lower jaws and teeth and believed to have existed from half a million to five million years ago. Its large jaw suggests a height and weight similar to the alleged Sasquatch. The problem is that many people assume that *Gigantopithecus* walked on its knuckles, like a gorilla, not on its two feet like a Sasquatch. But Krantz makes a good, if not conclusive, argument that based on the spread of its lower jaw, *Gigantopithecus* was actually an erect biped.

"If you change a gorilla to a vertical posture like a human," says Krantz, "and make the neck come straight down, one thing you have to do is spread the back of its lower jaw to make room for the neck. And, as you can see," he says holding a gorilla jaw in one hand and the *Gigantopithecus* jaw in the other, "the lower jaw of the *Gigantopithecus* spreads much more widely than the jaw of the gorilla." He concludes that *Gigantopithecus* was so much like the Sasquatch that he would assume *Gigantopithecus* "is still alive today."

Though Krantz's interest in Sasquatch tends to obscure his other contributions to anthropology, the creature is really just a chapter in his lifelong interest in human evolution. His doc-

toral dissertation at the University of Minnesota, boldly entitled "The Origin of Man," argued that early man rose above the
primates because he learned "persistence hunting." By stalk-
ing animals, Krantz contends, early man developed his concentration and his brain. He has since written two textbooks in anthropology, one on race, the other on evolution.

Whatever the subject matter, Krantz treats it in his own
creative and eccentric style. An early attempt to discover why
hairless foreheads evolved in early man had Krantz growing
his graying hair and beard for six months without telling his
colleagues anything of his experiment. He then donned a rub-
berized Neanderthal browridge so he could experience what it
would be like to be an early man in need of a haircut. "That
showed me why we have a retreating hairline," says Krantz. "It
kept the hair out of our faces."

Those colleagues who dismiss Krantz's Sasquatch theories by
no means dismiss his overall work in anthropology. Kelso calls
his work on human evolution "refreshing, novel and very imaginative." And Sherwood Washburn, professor emeritus of anthropology at the University of California, Berkeley, says of
Krantz, "He goes off on tangents that are not usually supporta-
ble, but he has been a very useful person in the profession. He
has made a lot of people think about a lot of things they
wouldn't have thought about otherwise."

But Krantz's knack for sometimes pursuing interests far removed from his own field of physical anthropology has proved
to be costly professionally. He is still an associate professor, although he has been eligible for full professorship for the past
six years. He explains that some of the faculty frown upon the
crossing of interdisciplinary lines, and cites as an example his
work showing that the dispersal of languages did not take place
through the migration of hunting people. "I was told four years
ago that I wasn't promoted to full professor because I had stuck
my nose into linguistics," he says. "I'm sure that now my Bigfoot work is a major part of the reason I continue to be passed up
for promotion."

The story of Krantz's search for Sasquatch actually provides
a persuasive argument for the existence of the creature. Sitting
in his small office, wearing jeans and a safari jacket and smok-

ing cigarettes, Krantz tells me that he has a long history of interest in unusual and unpopular ideas. "If someone says something is not true, my first reaction is: I wonder if it is?" says Krantz. "Of course, most of the time I find that it is not." But Sasquatch is different.

To Krantz, the diversity of reports suggested a perfectly straightforward biological phenomenon—a single species. And as a student of anthropology studying human origins at Berkeley in the early 1960s, Krantz felt that "to ignore the reports of the possibility of such a creature would be the height of stupidity." But at that time he was far from convinced about its existence. "If you had asked me then what odds I would place on whether the thing was real, I would have given you odds of about 10 to 1 against it," he says.

The breakthrough in Krantz's thinking came in the spring of 1970, a year after he had begun teaching at Washington State University. A few months earlier there had been a series of Sasquatch reports in northeastern Washington and several sets of tracks from a creature were photographed and recorded. What made these tracks so different from the thousands of Sasquatch footprints that had been observed and recorded in the past, however, was the distortion of the individual's right foot. Reasoning that the two bulges on the outside edge of the foot had probably been caused by some inflammation of the cartilage between the bones, Krantz was able to reconstruct the probable layout of the bones in the foot of this creature, which for obvious reasons has become known as "cripplefoot."

"Afterwards, when I compared the normal, though gigantic, left foot of the Sasquatch track to a seventeen-inch blow-up of an ordinary human foot," says Krantz, "I realized that this was not a typical human foot. The proportions were shifted. I was struck by the fact that the heel was relatively enormous, that the forepart of the foot, while big, was relatively much smaller than the human foot, and that the position of the ankle was set substantially farther forward. But that seemed perfectly reasonable. If an animal of this size was going to walk in step like a human, its leverage would have to be different."

Krantz then tackled the puzzle from a different angle. He calculated just how much the ankle would have to be moved forward on the basis of the Sasquatch's reported height and weight. Then he went back to his drawing of the bones on the cast of the Sasquatch footprint, measured the location of the ankle, and came up with the same figure. "That's when I decided the thing is real," says Krantz.

"There is no way a faker could have known how far forward to set that ankle," he says. "It took me a couple of months to work it out with the casts in hand, so you have to figure how much smarter a faker would've had to be. And I don't think there have been any genius anatomists floating around since Leonardo da Vinci. So either the animal is real or it's faked by a human being. Of those two choices, the real animal is ridiculous, the fake by the human impossible. Sherlock Holmes said 'When you have eliminated the impossible, whatever remains, however improbable, must be the truth.'"

Krantz now has a collection of some twenty casts of Sasquatch footprints and is convinced he can tell a real one from a fake. Sasquatch feet have flat arches, their heels are abnormally wide, the toes are short, and the forefoot is less tapered than the human foot. He also found, by making a fake pair of wooden feet, that a fake foot, when it rises, kicks up a little mound of dirt behind the toes in the footprint. Shoes or a bare foot kick up a mound of dirt back toward the middle of the foot. Krantz knows of two other traits that distinguish a real print, but he declines to identify them, fearing that hoaxers may use such information in the future.

The summer of 1970 brought forth more Sasquatch evidence. The handprints of one of these alleged animals were photographed, and plaster casts of them were made by a game guide in northeastern Washington State. The Sasquatch had apparently been digging in the ground and then put its hand down to stand up. "This palm is twice as wide as mine," says Krantz, holding the cast, "but it's half again as long. It goes with a footprint 19½ inches long. So the ratio between the hand and the foot is the same as it is in humans."

Krantz then points out the hand's most notable feature: Its thumb is turned in the same direction as all the rest of the fingers. A human thumb, by contrast, is opposable: It turns inward, toward the fingers. A primate with a non-opposable thumb, Krantz reasons, would have no muscles on its thenar pad, which is the elevated mound at the base of the thumb. The thenar area on such a primate would be flat, and, indeed, on the cast it's quite flat. "If it's a fake, the person had to know primate anatomy down to the last detail," he says. "That makes me convinced that this thing also has to be real."

But the story, like so many other Bigfoot stories, has a major kink in it. The game guide who discovered these handprints is believed to have subsequently faked a Sasquatch film. "I know a lot of people worry about that," replies Krantz, whose work on the handprint was published in 1971 in the journal *Northwest Anthropological Research Notes*. "The man is an expert nature photographer, but I know that he also happens to be quite uninformed about primate anatomy. I suspect that what happened was that after finding these handprints he thought he was going to bring one down or get a good movie of one. But after a while I think he got fed up and decided to fake it."

Though reports of the creature continued through the 1970s, no significant new piece of evidence came to light until June 10, 1982. On that day, Paul Freeman, a U.S. Forest Service patrolman of the Walla Walla district in Washington State, had been tracking elk when he encountered a hairy bipedal animal about eight feet tall. They looked at each other for thirty seconds from a distance of about sixty yards before the animal turned and walked away.

Stunned by the episode, Freeman immediately contacted his supervisors, who came and found a set of large footprints in the earth. The imprints were over an inch deep in fairly hard soil, indicating great body weight, and were located in an area closed to the public. Casts were made of these tracks and of others that Freeman and another patrolman found a week later just a few miles away from the original sighting. No animal had been observed at the second site, but the tracks indicated the presence of two individuals, perhaps a female and her offspring. One of the two was clearly the same individual Freeman had seen a week earlier, as both sets of tracks showed the same peculiar spreading out of the second toe of the left foot.

But it was the track from the other individual that intrigued Krantz. "It shows that the individual stepped on a stone," he says. "The foot spread out and hit firm ground on both sides of the stone, leaving a very deep indentation in the cast. Since there is no appreciable flexibility in the bones in that area of the foot, the sole of the foot must have had a very thick padding and itself been very flexible. I estimated that if it was a real foot, the pad had to be an inch to an inch and a half thick, made of fat and partitioned by connective tissue. I later found out that the gorilla has just such a pad on the base of its feet, but it's only three-quarters of an inch thick."

The feature that made the Walla Walla event so unique, however, was the discovery of dermal ridges on several tracks. These are the individual lines that are present on the fingers, toes, palms, and soles of all the higher primates. The ridges, spaced about half a millimeter apart, show bifurcations, terminations, and isolated short segments in various places—just the kind of variations that are seen in human prints. Also visible on the casts are what appear to be sweat pores.

"These details were directly imprinted on the side walls of the casts," says Krantz, "and thus could not have been made by a rigid structure with any combination of movements. A latex mold of real skin would have left expanded spaces between the ridges, and that is not the case here."

The casts were examined by more than a dozen fingerprint experts, from county deputies to the FBI, and by more than a half dozen anthropologists and zoologists, from the University of California to the Smithsonian. George Bonebrake, the former supervisor of the FBI's latent-fingerprint section, concludes that "there appear to be dermal ridges at various places on the cast of the footprint, but not enough to give an overall appearance or to base an opinion." Robert Olsen, a certified latent-print examiner for the Kansas Bureau of Investigation in Topeka, says he "could not detect that they were faked. If they were, it would have to be by somebody who had considerable knowledge about ridge details and anatomy, and it would have been a very time-consuming task." Tim White, a paleontologist at the University of California, Berkeley, says: "It's difficult to imagine how someone could fake those ridges. But I have to reserve judgment until Grover brings me a tooth or a bone." Ted Grand, a comparative anatomist associated with the Smithsonian's National Zoo, says: "Krantz is a very clever anatomist, but I didn't see anything in the tracks that compelled me to think that there are Sasquatch."

The reactions fell far short of Krantz's expectations. "It

seems to me," he says, "that if one brought in the skull of a Sasquatch, any twelve-year-old kid who had read an anthropology book could be absolutely competent to identify it. I don't think it takes any great knowledge or intelligence to accept the existence of something if you bring in the skeleton. But it takes a little bit of sleuthing and clear thinking to deduce from evidence like this what's behind it."

That has been done before, Krantz points out, with evidence far less convincing. When the footprints of two individuals were found in volcanic mud at the Laetoli site in east Africa a few years ago, they were immediately accepted by the National Geographic Society and Mary Leakey as evidence that man walked upright close to four million years ago. "Yet the quality of the footprints are nowhere near the quality of the prints we found at Walla Walla," says Krantz. "Unlike the Laetoli tracks, the Walla Walla tracks show separate toes, dermal ridges, and independent metatarsal movement."

While the lack of scientific acceptance has clearly disappointed Krantz, he understands the scientific community's reluctance. "We know that bigfoot data is 50 percent erroneous, and for the most part we don't know which 50 percent it is," says Krantz. "Science doesn't like to touch elusive data like that. And since there is a lot of fakery in this field, most scientists just assume that the rest of it is fake also. One anthropologist who looked at the Walla Walla tracks said to me if this was the only data you had on the Sasquatch, scientists would probably believe you. But because there is so much fakery going on, they are not going to pay much attention to this."

Krantz now realizes that only flesh and bone will ever establish the reality of the Sasquatch. "And the only reasonable way to get bones," he says, "is to go out and shoot one. That's okay because nothing indicates that it's human. No dependable Sasquatch report shows any sign of its using or making tools, communicating information by language, or being part of a social group. So it's an animal. And while some people advocate using a tranquilizer gun for humanitarian reasons, I think that's a mistake. Those guns have rotten accuracy, and since we've never gotten a Sasquatch before we don't know what drug to use, or how much, or where to hit him with it. Besides, whenever someone tries to tranquilize a new species, they end up killing ten to twenty in the process anyway."

If he had the funds, Krantz would hire five or ten big-game hunters with an interest in Sasquatch, each one assigned to an area of the Pacific Northwest familiar to the hunter, and where the creature has been sighted. He would give them $20,000 a year with a single requirement: Bring in a Sasquatch. Krantz believes that a big first prize and the ensuing publicity would probably be sufficient incentive to be the first, but to reduce the chances of cutthroat competition, he suggests that the rest of the hunters share a second prize the moment one of them brings in the Sasquatch. "I'm convinced they could do it in five years," says Krantz, who knows of three informal bigfoot hunts already underway.

Krantz thinks they have a good chance of success. He estimates that a viable breeding population of Sasquatch within the Pacific Northwest might number anywhere from two hundred to two thousand. "If there were more," says Krantz, "people would be seeing more of them, and they would be getting hit by cars and trains."

But if there are so many of them, then why haven't we found the bones of a Sasquatch already? "It would be surprising if bones were found," he says. "Hikers never come across the bones of wolves, badgers and coyotes unless they were killed by humans. If they die a natural death, they hide. It's not normal to find the remains of large, uncommon animals. I have yet to find a hunter or game guide who has found a bear that died a natural death."

Despite their apparent numbers, however, the Sasquatch are almost always seen singly. "That's very typical of bear behavior," says Krantz, "every individual for him or herself. But that's not too surprising. For a primate living in a primarily temperate forest where the concentration of food is not very great, a large herd of them would not be effective. But of course if they are so thinly spread, I wondered for some time how would they locate each other, especially for mating purposes. Well, I can't answer that for sure, but the vocalizations that have been reported, the loud screams, might well be a mechanism for locating one another."

As far as diet is concerned, the Sasquatch have been observed picking up fruits and vegetables and sometimes stealing food from people. This suggests to Krantz that, like bears, the Sasquatch are primarily vegetarians and opportunistic carnivores.

But unlike bears, who sack out around midnight and get up late in the morning, the Sasquatch appear to be nocturnal animals, as they are most often seen between midnight and dawn. "Since bears and Sasquatch are almost direct competitors for all resources," says Krantz, "it's not surprising to see that the bears and the Sasquatch have divided up the day between them to keep out of each other's way."

Krantz has a long history of sticking his neck out for his work. "So far," he boasts, "my track record is no failures, a lot of uncertainties and a few successes." He is convinced that he will be proven right on the Sasquatch as well, but for the moment he is nearly alone in the scientific community to state such a belief openly. "Others are scared for their reputations and their jobs," says Krantz, standing up and putting on his worn blue cap with its Peking Man pin. "But I prefer honesty to tact. That's one of my character flaws."

ULTIMATE SECRET

In the early morning of December 27, 1980, two security patrol-men stationed at the American Air Force Base at Bentwaters, England saw unusual lights in the nearby Rendlesham Forest. Thinking that an aircraft might have crashed, they asked for and received permission to investigate. A third patrolman joined them and they proceeded on foot.

What happened then is described in an official document of the 81st Combat Support Group, dated January 13, 1981, en-titled "Unexplained Lights," and signed by the Deputy Base Commander, Lt. Col. Halt. The document reads:

"The individuals reported seeing a strange glowing object in the forest. The object was described as being metallic in appear-ance and triangular in shape, approximately two to three meters across the base and approximately two meters high. It illuminated the entire forest with a white light. The object itself had a pulsating red light on top with a bank(s) of blue lights un-derneath. The object was hovering or on legs. As the patrolmen approached the object, it maneuvered through the trees and disappeared. At this time the animals on a nearby farm went into a frenzy. . . ."

The next day, the reports continues, "three depressions one and one-half inches deep and seven inches in diameter were found where the object had been sighted on the ground." When the area was checked for radiation the following night, they found peak readings "in the three depressions and near the cen-ter of the triangle formed by the depressions." More strange lights were seen in the area that night.

What happened at Bentwaters in 1980? No other government documents are available on the incident, but some of those who claim to have been there that night and on subsequent nights give accounts of high Air Force personnel involved with a metallic craft and mysterious entities in a clearing in the Rendlesham Forest. Whatever really happened at Bentwaters, we know for certain that the Air Force was involved and their own paperwork proves it.

Despite official pronouncements for decades that UFOs were nothing more than misidentified aerial objects and as such were no cause for alarm, declassified Government records now indicate that, ever since UFOs made their appearance in our skies in the 1940s, the phenomenon has aroused much serious behind-the-scenes concern in official circles. Details of the intelligence community's protracted obsession with the subject of UFOs have now emerged with the release of long-withheld Government documents obtained through the Freedom of Information Act (FOIA). Though these papers fail to resolve the UFO enigma, they do dispel many popular notions about the UFO controversy, as well as give substance to a number of others.

Official records now available appear to put to rest doubts that the Government knew more about UFOs than it has claimed over the past four decades. From the start, it has been convinced that most UFO sightings could be explained in terms of misidentified balloons, cloud formations, airplanes, ball lightning, meteors and other natural phenomenon. But the documents also show that the Government remains perplexed about UFOs. Do they pose a threat to national security? Are they just a funny-looking cover for an airborne Soviet presence? Even the possibility that these unknowns could be evidence of extraterrestrial visitations has been given serious attention in Government circles.

While official interest in UFOs has long been thought to be strictly the concern of the Air Force, the bulk of whose records have been open to public view for more than a decade, the documents on UFOs that have been released under the FOIA indicate otherwise. The Departments of the Army, Navy, State and Defense, and the Defense Intelligence Agency, the National Security Agency, the Joint Chiefs of Staff, the FBI, the CIA, and even the Atomic Energy Commission produced UFO records over the years. Many of these agencies still do, and many of their documents remain classified. The CIA is still withholding more than fifty documents, the National Security Agency more than one hundred.

The monumental task of unearthing these records from a bureaucracy that has denied their existence for years can be traced to the efforts of a handful of inquisitive individuals who, armed with the FOIA, set off in the mid-1970s on a paper chase of U.S. Government documents on UFOs. They include Bruce Maccabee, a physicist working for the Navy, who obtained the release of more than a thousand pages of FBI documents on UFOs; Todd Zechel; Brad Sparks; Larry Bryant; Robert Todd; and Peter Gersten, a New York attorney, whose 1977 civil action against the CIA, produced almost a thousand pages of UFO-related memos, reports and correspondence that attest to the agency's long involvement in the matter. This documentary evidence adds a new dimension to what has been known of the Government's involvement with UFOs up until this point (see *The UFO Controversy in America* by David Michael Jacobs and *Clear Intent* by Lawrence Fawcett and Barry Greenwood).

Here then is a brief history of the modern UFO controversy:

The first sighting to be labeled a "flying saucer" by the press occurred on June 24, 1947, when an Idaho businessman flying his plane near Mt. Rainier observed nine disc-shaped objects making undulating motions "like a saucer skipping over water." But as early as World War II, Allied bomber pilots had told of "balls of light" that followed their flights over Japan and Germany. Rumor had it that the objects were enemy secret weapons, but as the objects showed no hostility, many servicemen believed them to be psychological warfare devices sent aloft to unnerve American pilots. A U.S. Eighth Army investigation concluded that they were the product of "mass hallucination."

When Scandinavians reported cigar-shaped objects in 1946, U.S. Army intelligence suspected that the Russians had developed a secret weapon with the help of German scientists from Peenemunde. The CIA, then known as the Central Intelligence Group, secretly began keeping tabs on the subject.

When the unknown objects returned to the skies, this time

over the United States in the summer of 1947, the Army Air Force set out to determine what the objects were. Within weeks, Brig. Gen. George Schulgen of Army Air Corps Intelligence requested the FBI's assistance "in locating and questioning the individuals who first sighted the so-called flying discs . . . ." Undoubtedly swayed by flaring cold war tensions, Schulgen feared that "the first reported sightings might have been by individuals of Communist sympathies with the view to causing hysteria and fear of a secret Russian weapon." J. Edgar Hoover agreed to cooperate but insisted that the bureau have "full access to discs recovered."

The Air Force's behind-the-scenes interest contrasted sharply with its public stance that the objects were products of misidentifications and an imaginative populace. A security lid was imposed on the subject in July 1947, hiding a potentially "embarrassing situation" the following month, when both the Air Force and the FBI began suspecting they might actually be investigating our own secret weapons. High-level reassurances were obtained that this was not so.

By the end of the summer, the FBI had "failed to reveal any indication of subversive individuals being involved in any of the reported sightings." A RESTRICTED Army letter that found its way to Hoover's desk said that the bureau's services actually had been enlisted to relieve the Air Force "of the task of tracking down all the many instances which turned out to be ashcan covers, toilet seats and whatnot." FBI personnel had begun to suspect that the bureau was "merely playing bird-dog for the Army." Incensed, Hoover moved quickly to discontinue the bureau's UFO investigations.

In September of that year, the Commanding General of the Army Air Force received a letter from the Army Chief of Staff Lieut. Gen. Nathan Twining, saying that "the phenomenon reported is of something real and not visionary or fictitious," that the objects appeared to be disc-shaped, "as large as man-made aircraft," and "controlled either manually, automatically or remotely." At Twining's request, a permanent project, code named Sign and classified RESTRICTED, was established in December of 1947.

Sign failed to find any evidence that the objects were Soviet secret weapons and before long submitted an unofficial "Estimate of the Situation," classified TOP SECRET, which indicated that UFOs were of interplanetary origin. The estimate eventually reached Air Force Chief of Staff Gen. Hoyt Vandenberg, who rejected it for lack of proof. Sign's inconclusive final report remained classified for the next twelve years.

The CIA's Office of Scientific Intelligence (OSI) took note of the Sign report. Flying discs would probably turn out to be another "sea serpent," an OSI officer believed, but should be investigated on the "remote possibility that they may be interplanetary or foreign aircraft." Meanwhile, the FBI advised its agents that the flying discs might be Russian man-made missiles, and Hoover instructed his agents to follow the new Air Force UFO reporting procedures should anyone volunteer UFO information. For the most part, this passive stance—referring UFO reports to the Air Force without action by the Bureau—sums up the extent of the FBI's investigations to this day.

Perhaps the most intriguing document in FBI files, however, is dated March 22, 1950. This memo to Hoover from a bureau agent notes that the Air Force had recovered three flying saucers in New Mexico. "They were described as being circular in shape with raised centers, approximately fifty feet in diameter," the agent wrote. "Each one was occupied by three bodies of human shape but only three feet tall, dressed in metallic cloth of a very fine texture." More than thirty years later, this document would inspire Larry Bryant of Citizens Against UFO Secrecy (CAUS) to file a petition for a "Writ of Habeas Corpus Extraterrestrial," claiming that the Air Force maintained custody over one or more occupants, dead or alive, of crashed flying saucers. A U.S. District Court judge in Washington, D.C. dismissed the case, however, on the grounds that the court had no jurisdiction over the case and that the plaintiff had no authority to represent the alleged creatures.

After Sign, the Air Force continued to collect UFO data under the code name Grudge. This six-month project found no evidence of foreign scientific development and therefore no direct threat to national security. It did, however, stress that the reported sightings could be dangerous. "There are indications that the planned release of related psychological propaganda would cause a form of mass hysteria," the report stated. A press release following the termination of Grudge allowed the public to believe that the Air Force was no longer interested in UFOs. But the Air Force continued to collect reports through normal intelligence channels until the dramatic sighting of a UFO at the Army Signal Corps radar center in Fort Monmouth, N.J. in 1951 led to the reactivation of Grudge. The Air Force project was renamed Blue Book in 1952, a year that saw a record number of UFO reports.

The situation got out of hand that summer. On the morning of July 28th, the *Washington Post* revealed that UFOs had been tracked on radar at Washington National Airport, the second such incident in a week. Reporters stormed Air Force headquarters in the Pentagon, where switchboards were jammed for days with UFO inquiries. Military installations across the country handled such a volume of reports that "regular intelligence work had been affected," reported the *New York Times*.

These events prompted action at CIA headquarters, apparently at a request "from the Hill." From the start, the agency's involvement was to be kept secret. An August 1st CIA memo recommended that "no indication of CIA interest or concern reach the press or public, in view of their probable alarmist tendencies to accept such interest as 'confirmatory' of the soundness of 'unpublished facts' in the hands of the U.S. Government."

The CIA's Office of Scientific Intelligence (OSI) found that the Air Force's investigation of the UFO phenomenon was not sufficiently rigorous to determine the exact nature of the objects in the sky. Nor did the Air Force deal adequately with the potential danger of UFO-induced mass hysteria, or the fact that our air vulnerability was being seriously affected by the UFO problem. OSI chief H. Marshall Chadwell thought that our nation's defenses were running the increasing risk of false alert and, worse yet, "of falsely identifying the real as phantom." He suggested that a national policy be established "as to what should be told the public" and, furthermore, that immediate steps be taken to improve our current visual and electronic identification techniques so that "instant positive identification of enemy planes or missiles can be made."

Ever vigilant, the CIA was keeping an eye on the possibility that UFOs could be of Soviet origin. Checking with the Agency's Foreign Broadcast Information Division, they uncovered no mention of flying saucers in the Soviet Union. The only Soviet reference to UFOs had appeared in the *New York Times,* where Soviet foreign minister Gromyko joked about the discs coming from Soviet discus throwers practicing for the Olympics. Despite the apparent Soviet official policy of silence, a review by OSI did "not lead to the conclusion that the saucers are USSR created or controlled." Nevertheless, the CIA's interest in foreign sightings and opinions regarding UFOs, particularly those in the Soviet Union, continues to this day. "The agency's interest," says Katherine Pherson, a public-affairs officer for the CIA, "lies in its responsibility to forewarn principally of the possibility that a foreign power might develop a new weapons system that might exhibit phenomena that some might categorize as a UFO."

By the winter of 1952, Chadwell had drafted a National Security Council proposal calling for a program to solve the problem of instant positive identification of UFOs. In a memo that accompanied the proposal, Chadwell urged that the reports be given "immediate attention." He thought that "sightings of unexplained objects at great altitudes and traveling at high speeds in the vicinity of major U.S. defense installations are of such nature that they are not attributable to natural phenomena or known types of aerial vehicles." He said that OSI was proceeding with the establishment of a consulting group "of sufficient competence and stature to . . . convince the responsible authorities in the community that immediate research and development on this subject must be undertaken."

But CIA Director Gen. Walter B. Smith's interest apparently lay elsewhere. In a letter to the Director of the Psychological Strategy Board, he expressed a desire to discuss "the possible offensive and defensive utilization of these phenomena for psychological warfare purposes." Only later, after an order from the Intelligence Advisory Committee, did Director Smith authorize recruiting an advisory committee of outside consultants.

The scientific panel met for four days beginning January 14, 1953. Chaired by Dr. H. P. Robertson, an expert in physics and weapons systems, the panel essentially bestowed the scientific seal of approval on previously established official policy regarding UFOs. The distinguished panelists felt that all the sightings could be identified once all the data were available for a proper evaluation—in other words, the phenomena, according to the panel's report, were not "beyond the domain of present knowledge of physical sciences." Neither did the panelists find UFOs to be a direct threat to national security, though they believed that the volume of UFO reports could clog military intelligence channels, precipitate panic and lead defense personnel to ignore real indications of hostile action. The panel worried about Soviet manipulation of the phenomenon; that the reports could make the public vulnerable to "possible enemy psychological warfare." The real danger, they concluded, was the reports themselves.

Fearing that the myth of UFOs might lead to inappropriate actions by the American public, the panelists decided that a "broad educational program integrating efforts of all concerned agencies" must be undertaken. They sought to strip UFOs of their "aura of mystery" through this program of "training and 'debunking.'" The program would result in the "proper recognition of unusually illuminated objects" and in a "reduction in public interest in 'flying saucers.'" The panelists recommended that their mass-media program have as its advisers psychologists familiar with mass psychology and advertising experts, while Walt Disney Inc. animated cartoons and such personalities as Arthur Godfrey would help in the educational drive. To insure complete control over the situation, the panel members suggested that flying saucer groups be "watched because of their potentially great influence on mass thinking if widespread sightings should occur. The apparent irresponsibility and the possible use of such groups for subversive purposes should be kept in mind."

The panel's recommendations called for nothing less than the domestic manipulation of public attitudes. Whether these proposals were acted upon, the CIA will not say. But the report was circulated among the top brass at the Air Technical Intelligence Center, the CIA's Board of National Estimates, the CIA's bureau chiefs, the Secretary of Defense, the chairman of the National Security Resources Board, and the director of the Federal Civil Defense Administration, who eventually sent a representative to meet with CIA officials in order to "implement the appropriate aspets of the Panel's Report as applicable to Civil Defense."

Certainly the conduct of the Air Force in the UFO controversy changed in 1953. Until its termination in 1969, Blue Book seemed to concentrate more on the public relations problem generated by UFO reports than on the nature of the phenomenon itself. Blue Book managed to reduce the volume of reports that remained unidentified after investigation from 17 percent for the period preceding 1953, to 6 percent afterward, though twice as many reports were recorded between 1953 and 1969. That process of minimizing the pesky residue of unknowns began on the Air Force's own doorstep. In August of 1953, the Air Force issued Regulation 200-2, which streamlined UFO reporting procedures and also prohibited the public release of any information about a sighting unless the sighting was positively identified.

But the Government's efforts in the 1950s and 1960s to squelch public apprehension over UFOs went beyond debunking and even touched the fiber of constitutionally protected free speech. According to historian David Michael Jacobs, in 1953 the Air Force pressured *Look* magazine into publishing disclaimers throughout an article by retired Maj. Donald E. Keyhoe entitled "Flying Saucers From Outer Space." Then again, in 1965, the Army—in a prepublication review—denied clearance for a UFO-related article by one of its employees, Larry Bryant, a technical writer, until he took the issue to court.

Meanwhile, the CIA and the FBI proceeded routinely in the surveillance of UFO organizations and UFO enthusiasts. People with UFO interests were checked out by the FBI at the request of the CIA, the Air Force, or private citizens inquiring about possible subversive activities. But none caused as much consternation as the case of Major Keyhoe and the organization he directed, the National Investigations Committee on Aerial Phenomena (NICAP).

The CIA appears to have had a protracted interest in NICAP, which was founded in 1956 and utilized by Keyhoe as an organizational tool for challenging the alleged Air Force cover-up on UFOs. Both the CIA and the Air Force were upset by NICAP's wide-ranging influence. Its prestigious board of directors included, among others, Vice Adm. Roscoe Hillenkoetter, the first CIA director (1947–1950). "The Air Force representatives believe that much of the trouble ... with Major Keyhoe ...

could be alleviated," states a CIA memo dated May 16, 1958, "if the Major did not have such important personages as Vice Admiral R. H. Hillenkoetter, U. S. N. (Ret.) . . . on the board . . . ." The Air Force suggested that if the Admiral were shown the SECRET panel report he might understand and take "appropriate actions." Whether or not the Air Force got through to the Admiral, Hillenkoetter resigned from NICAP in 1961. The CIA's interest in NICAP continued through the 1970s when the UFO organization became so ineffective that it was dissolved.

Mounting discontent from members of the media, Congress and the scientific community compelled the Air Force in 1966 to commission an eighteen-month scientific study of UFOs under the direction of Edward Condon, professor of physics at the University of Colorado. The politically expedient study, in which one-third of the ninety-one cases examined remained unidentified, reiterated official policy with one novel twist: UFOs "educationally harmed" schoolchildren who were allowed to use science study time to read books and magazine articles about UFOs. Condon wanted techers to withhold credit from any student UFO project. The Air Force took the cue and disbanded Project Blue Book in 1969.

Blue Book's true nature as well as the Air Force's continuing interest in UFOs was revealed many years later when an Air Force memo from Brig. Gen. C. H. Bolender, dated Oct. 20, 1969, was released. Replying to concern over the upcoming termination of Blue Book, Bolender commented that Project Blue Book had never received those reports that affected national security anyway. "Reports of unidentified flying objects which could affect national security are made in accordance with JANAP 146 or Air Force Manual 55–11, and are not part of the Blue Book system. . . . as already stated, reports of UFOs which could affect national security would continue to be handled through the standard Air Force procedures designed for this purpose."

One of the more fascinating of all the Government UFO documents is a National Security Agency (NSA) draft report, dated 1968, which may have been prepared at the Condon Committee's request. It is entitled "UFO Hypothesis and Human Survival Questions." In the report, a NSA analyst considered some of the implications suggested by the primary UFO hypothesis. If

UFOs are hoaxes, the analyst wrote, "then a human mental aberration of alarming proportions would appear to be developing. Such an aberration would seem to have serious implications for nations equipped with nuclear toys—and should require immediate and careful study by scientists."

Though "the evidence seems to argue strongly against all UFOs being hallucinations," the analyst continued, if indeed they are hallucinations, then "the psychological implications for man would certainly bring into strong question his ability to distinguish reality from fantasy." If UFOs are natural phenomenon, the analyst said, then "the capability of air warning systems to correctly diagnose an attack situation is open to serious question." He also stated that "all UFOs should be carefully scrutinized to ferret-out. . .enemy (or 'friendly') projects," just in case they are secret Earth projects.

The NSA analyst concluded by considering the possibility that UFOs might be related to extraterrestrial intelligence. He said that if certain eminent scientists are to be believed, then this possibility cannot be dismissed. And if they are extraterrestrial, he believed that they would be our technological superiors. History has shown, said the analyst, that when this happens the inferior people are normally subjected to physical conquest, causing a loss of cultural and national identity. For these reasons, he suggested that, "a little more of. . .[a] survival attitude is called for in dealing with the UFO problem."

What happened in the decade that followed seems to bear him out. Government documents on UFOs indicate that an advanced technology seems to be involved, that UFOs sometimes pose a threat to national security, and that military and intelligence agencies still express concern over the phenomenon, despite official pronouncements to the contrary.

On September 8, 1973, according to a Department of the Army document, two military policemen at Hunter Army Airfield in Georgia "noticed an 'object' traveling at what appeared to them to be a high rate of speed traveling east to west at approximately two thousand feet altitude and crossing the post perimeter. Approximately ten minutes later they resighted the 'object' when it appeared at 'treetop' level and made an apparent dive at their vehicle seemingly just missing their vehicle." The object, which made "no noise" while hovering for about fifteen minutes in front of them, was "round or oval in shape" and "between thirty-five and seventy-five feet across."

Two years later, in March of 1975, a Department of State message reported that "responsible people" had observed "strange machines" maneuvering in Algerian airspace. The light, which was so bright as to obscure its shape, was tracked first on radar and then seen to "land and take off."

Then just six months later, a UFO flap engulfed U.S. military bases. A Defense Department message on "Suspicious Unknown Air Activity" and dated Nov. 11, 1975, reads: "Since 28 Oct 75 numerous reports of suspicious objects have been received at the NORAD COC (North American Air Defense Combat Operations Center). Reliable military personnel at Loring AFB (Air Force Base), Maine, Wurtsmith AFB, Michigan, Malmstrom AFB, (Montana), Minot AFB, (North Dakota), and Canadian Forces Station, Falconbridge, Ontario, Canada, have visually sighted suspicious objects."

"Objects at Loring and Wurtsmith were characterized to be helicopters. Missile site personnel, security alert teams and Air Defense personnel at Malmstrom Montana report objects which sounded like a jet aircraft. FAA advised 'There were no jet aircraft in the vicinity.' Malmstrom search and height finder radars carried the object between 9,000 ft and 15,000 ft at a speed of seven knots. . . . F-106s scrambled from Malmstrom could not make contact due to darkness and low altitude. Site personnel reported the objects as low as 200 ft and said that as the interceptors approached the lights went out. After the interceptors had passed the lights came on again. One hour after the F-106s returned to base, missile site personnel reported the objects increased to a high speed, raised in altitude and could not be discerned from the stars. . . ."

"I have expressed my concern to SAFOI [Air Force Information Office] that we come up soonest with a proposed answer to queries from the press to prevent overreaction by the public to reports by the media that may be blown out of proportion. To date efforts by Air Guard helicopters, SAC [Strategic Air Command] helicopters and NORAD F-106s have failed to produce positive ID."

Numerous daily updates kept the Joint Chiefs of Staff informed of these incursions by UFOs. Representatives of the Defense Intelligence Agency and the National Security Agency as well as a handful of other Government desks received copies of the National Military Command Center's reports on the incidents. One report said that an unidentified object "demonstrated a clear intent in the weapons storage area." Though Air Force records show that the CIA was notified several times of these penetrations over nuclear missile and bomber bases, the agency has acknowledged only one such notification. Subsequent investigations by the Air Force into the sightings at Loring Air Force Base, Maine, where the remarkable series of events began, did not reveal a cause for the sightings.

Whatever the objects were, the incidents created quite a stir. The Air Force implemented "Security Option 3" at the northern tier bases, according to an Air Force Security Police message, because of unidentified objects "flying/hovering over priority A restricted areas." NORAD also instituted a new set of reporting procedures as a result of these sightings. All those inquiring from the media and public, says a NORAD document entitled "Replies to UFO Reports," should be told that the Air Force "no longer investigates UFO reports" and "has no official interest in UFOs." The document then goes on to say that "all UFO/unknown object information no matter what the source might be—civilian or military" were to be submitted to the National Combat Operations Center.

The following year, 1976, saw another flap of military-related UFO incidents. On January 21st, according to a National Military Command Center (NMCC) memo signed by Rear Admiral J.B. Morin, security police observed two UFOs near the flight line at Canon Air Force Base in New Mexico. The objects were "25 yards in diameter, gold or silver in color with a blue light on top, hole in the middle and red light on bottom."

Six months later, on July 30th, UFOs were seen in the vicinity of Fort Ritchie, Maryland by both civilian and military personnel, according to another NMCC memo. One of the three oblong objects was seen "over the ammo storage area at 100-200 yards altitude." A month later in Tunisia "phenomena completely unexplainable" were seen and tracked on radar over the space of several nights. The objects, according to the document, could both travel at "high speeds" or slowly enough to "hover."

One of the most fascinating of all the government UFO documents tells of an extraordinary episode that took place on September 19, 1976 over Iran. The Defense Intelligence Agency (DIA) message reports that American-made Iranian jets encountered several UFOs which caused one jet to lose "all instrumentation and communications." The primary object, which appeared to be the size of a 707 tanker on radar, had "flashing strobe lights arranged in a rectangular pattern and alternating blue, green, red and orange in color." As the pursuit by the F-4 jets continued "another brightly lighted object, estimated to be one half to one third the apparent size of the moon, came out of the original object. This second object headed straight toward the F-4 at a very fast rate of speed. The pilot attempted to fire an AIM-9 missile at the object but at that instant his weapons control panel went off and he lost all communications."

The DIA, in its evaluation of the incident, called it "an outstanding UFO report." The object, the report stated, "was seen by multiple witnesses from different locations. . .and viewpoints (both airborne and from the ground). The credibility of many of the witnesses was high. . . . Visual sightings were confirmed by radar. Similar electromagnetic effects (EME) were reported by three separate aircraft. There were physiological effects on some members. . . . [and] an inordinate amount of maneuverability was displayed by the UFOs."

Two years later, according to a Naval Air Station Message Report, on May 14, 1978, civilians at the Pinecastle range in Jacksonville, Florida reported seeing "an object about 50-60 feet in diameter" passing over them "at tree-top level." The object was observed on radar for about an hour before moving across the scope at a high rate of speed—"400 to 500 knots." It then "reversed direction" and "practically stopped moving." Eight Navy personnel watched the object's red, green and white lights from the control tower for over an hour.

The following year, UFOs appeared over Kuwait, according to a State Department message dated January 29, 1979. One UFO, which appeared over the northern oil fields, "seemingly did strange things" to the automatic pumping equipment. The UFO's appearance apparently caused the automatic pumping equipment to shut down, and though the system could normally only be restarted manually, it started up again automatically when the UFO "vanished."

A Department of Defense Joint Chief of Staff message, dated June 3, 1980 reported that UFOs were seen on two different occasions near a Peruvian Air Force (PAF) Base in the southern part of the country. "The PAF tried to intercept and destroy the UFO but without success," says the report. Six months later, in December, UFOs were reported on the Czechoslovakian border, according to a U.S. Army cable obtained from the CIA.

Though the Air Force admits to nothing more than a "transitory interest" in the phenomenon these days, military directives still exist for reporting UFOs. Likewise, the CIA's interest appears passive. "There is no program to actively collect information on UFOs," says CIA spokesman Pherson. But the agency's interest cannot be denied, as two 1976 memos reveal.

The first, dated April 26th, states: "It does not seem that the Government has any formal program in progress for the identification/solution of the UFO phenomenon. Dr. [name deleted] feels that the efforts of independent researchers, [phrase deleted], are vital for further progress in this area. At the present time, there are offices and personnel within the agency who are monitoring the UFO phenomenon, but again, this is not currently on an official basis."

Another memo, dated July 14th, and routed to the deputy chief in the Office of Development and Engineering, reads: "As you may recall, I mentioned my own interest in the subject as well as the fact that DCD [Domestic Collection Division] has been receiving material from many of our S&T [Science and Technology] sources who are presently conducting related research. These scientists include some who have been associated with the Agency for years and whose credentials remove them from the 'nut' variety."

The final chapter of the UFO story has yet to be written. Some believe it will tell of the story of a popular fantasy. Others are convinced it will tell the story of contact with extraterrestrial intelligence and the great cover-up that followed. That is why they call it the ultimate secret.

GLOWING BIRDS
AND OTHER ANOMALIES

Phosphorescent night herons, hens shining like balls of white fire, barn owls that emit a pale yellow glow visible four hundred yards off—such sightings of luminous birds have been published, but not fully explained, in scientific literature from Pliny's *Historia Naturalis* to recent reports of the U.S. Fish and Wildlife Service. These avian anomalies and thousands of other unexplained observations, embarrassing deviations and paradigm-shattering discoveries from the dark corners of science might have remained buried in obscure journals if they hadn't been rescued by William Corliss, a fifty-seven-year-old physicist turned stalker of paradoxical data.

Like a one-man fact factory, Corliss has spent the past dozen years poring through more than five thousand scientific journals, and gleaning from them a wide assortment of neglected data from many disciplines: geology, biology, archaeology, astronomy, geophysics and psychology. Thus far, he has reprinted verbatim the most noteworthy of those items in a series of ten loose-leaf binders, six hefty hardbacks, and four detailed catalogs. This massive assemblage of data is part of what Corliss calls the Sourcebook Project.

The entire Sourcebook Project, he estimates, represents about two thousand well-defined phenomena and anomalies that are not completely explained by current theories and hypotheses. Of course, not all these anomalies are of equal significance to science. Glowing birds are certainly not as important as anomalies challenging Einstein's theories or the Big Bang. But all the entries in Corliss's collection have one characteristic in common: they illustrate the notion that the hard facts of science are far more tentative and provisional than we have been led to believe.

"It is this very strangeness of nature that makes science engrossing," says Dr. Lewis Thomas, chancellor of the Memorial Sloan-Kettering Cancer Center. Thomas points out what he believes is a serious flaw in the way science is being taught these days: its portrayal as a vast array of hard facts to be learned as fundamentals. Instead, says Thomas, we should leave "the fundamentals, the so-called basics, aside for a while, and concentrate the attention of all students on the things that are not known.

"We do not understand much of anything," he admits, "from the episode we rather dismissively, and I think defensively, choose to call the Big Bang, all the way down to the particles in the atoms of a bacterial cell. We have a wilderness of mystery to make our way through in the centuries ahead." He suggests that a new set of courses be designed to deal systematically with the unknown in science.

Corliss's Sourcebooks could well be the texts for such a course, even though the vast majority of Sourcebook entries are low-priority puzzles and curiosities. Confirming the existence of the Loch Ness monster, for example, would scarcely cause a ripple in zoology. Why? Because the reappearance of a supposedly extinct creature would require no readjustment of scientific principles. But as many as a third of the phenomena might require such a readjustment, according to Corliss, and of these about fifty might prove to be truly Earth-shaking.

One anomaly with paradigm-shattering potential concerns an experiment that illustrates the astonishing amount of control the mind appears to have over the body. For over a century such respected scientific journals as the *Psychological Bulletin, Lancet,* and the *American Journal of Psychiatry* have reported experiments in which blisters have been produced on the skin through hypnotic suggestion. In one case, the distinguished psychiatrist Montague Ullman described how a twenty-seven-year-old Swiss soldier was told, during a hypnotic session, that fever blisters would form around the right corner of his lower lip within twenty-four hours. At the start of the session, the soldier showed no evidence of any respiratory infection or incipient lesions about the mouth. He was then kept under observation for twenty-four hours. By the next morning, the soldier had developed "multiple small blisters about the lower lip in the right-hand corner."

Equally controversial are the reports of a link between the positions of the planets and cycles of solar activity. The Sourcebook references indicate that the subject has been tossed about in mainstream scientific literature for more than a century. Some scientists claim to have found a correlation between the height of the tide raised on the sun by various planetary alignments and the dates of sunspot maxima and minima. Yet no effect of gravity or any other force produced by the planets seems powerful enough to influence the sun in such a way.

Anomalies like these tend to annoy the orthodox scientist. "Few things are harder to put up with than the annoyance of a good example," said Mark Twain. Orthodox science prefers to view itself as a logical, virtually errorless march toward immutable truth. Yet surrounding the accredited facts of every science, said Williams James, the father of American psychology, "floats a sort of dust-cloud of exceptional observations, of occurrences minute and irregular and seldom met with, which it always proves more easy to ignore than to attend to."

Corliss has certainly been attending to them, and he is not alone these days. "I think there is more material appearing now on anomalies in the scientific literature than ever before," he reports.

This dealer in neglected scientific data brings solid authority to his present pursuit. After receiving degrees in physics from Rensselaer Polytechnic Institute and the University of Colorado, he worked for ten years as a physicist in industry. His fascination with scientific curiosities, however, ultimately led him to the serious and systematic collection of phenomena that refuse to fit the picture of reality provided by conventional wisdom and established science.

Known in some quarters as anomalistics, this interdisciplinary field of research is less than a century old. The term itself was coined just a decade ago by Roger Wescott, a professor of anthropology and linguistics at Drew University in New Jersey. Wescott considers John Haldane, the British geneticist, to be the precursory genius of anomalistics. Haldane was fond of commenting on "the inexhaustible queerness of things" and is said to have observed that "the universe is not only stranger than we imagine but stranger than we *can* imagine."

The title of founder of anomalistics, however, belongs to Charles Fort, an independently wealthy American journalist who spent most of his life (1874-1936) gathering and classifying reports that did not fit accepted scientific theory. He recognized, for instance, the validity of "stones falling from the sky" long before scientists of the day stopped laughing and acknowledged the existence of meteorites.

Unlike Fort, who always made a point of showing up the establishment, Corliss holds no grudge against science, and it seems that most scientists are quite tolerant of him. (Academics account for a quarter of all Sourcebook Project sales, libraries for half.) Certainly his project has not raised the kind of antagonism that once greeted the works of Immanuel Velikovsky and Erich von Daniken. Any such attack would surely be unjustified, for nearly all of the material in the Sourcebook Project is drawn from the literature of science itself.

Corliss was put on the trail of the scientific anomaly thirty years ago, when he picked up a second-hand copy of George McCready Price's *Evolutionary Geology and the New Catastrophism.* He later discovered that there were many more puzzling things in geology than Price had ever dreamed of, and one product of that discovery is the Sourcebook Project volume entitled *Unknown Earth.* This handbook of geological enigmas contains evidence that strains the theory of continental drift, a favorite of contemporary geologists.

Continental drift may be an oversimplification of the complex structural conditions of the Earth's crust, according to one *Unknown Earth* item, a reprint of a 1967 article by Victor Oppenheim in the *American Association of Petroleum Geologists Bulletin.* Numerous observations of the continents and ocean floors indicate that continental masses were probably not displaced over thousands of miles, as continental drift would have us believe. A more plausible explanation for the separation of continental masses, Oppenheim suggests, may be found in the pattern of global fracture zones circling the Earth, across the Atlantic, Pacific and Indian ocean floors. These zones suggest that the positions of the continents are related to an expansion of the Earth's crust.

Among the bones of contention that appear in the pages of

the Sourcebook volume called *Mysterious Universe* are doubts about the Big Bang, the question of possible biological material in meteorites, the reported changes in the gravitational constant—even observations of phantom moons orbiting the Earth. For close to a century, astronomers around the world have reported seeing these extra moons. The German astronomer Dr. G. Waltemath announced in the late 1890s that he had discovered not only a second moon but a whole system of midget moons around the Earth. In 1960, a Polish astronomer, Dr. K. Kordylewski, reported the discovery of two faint, cloudlike objects circling the Earth at the same distance as the moon. Astronomer John Bagby has claimed several observations that suggest that the Earth has at least ten natural moonlets, which broke off from a larger parent body in 1955.

Throughout the volume, Corliss parades a wealth of older astronomical observations that have yet to be recognized. "I feel sure that a lot of observations are legitimate and have reasonable explanations," says Corliss, "but they are now discarded or being ignored because no theory exists to explain them. I think that an eyewitness is an eyewitness. Just because some of them lived a hundred years ago or so doesn't make them any less qualified."

Geophysics has not been spared the Corliss treatment, and in his *Handbook of Unusual Natural Phenomena* the Earth and the heavens reveal themselves as extraordinary showmen. In July 1964, a ship's crew reported the appearance of a series of pale blue, chartreuse and magenta concentric rings on the horizon where the sun had set. A shower of sand eels fell on Handon, England, in 1918; Peruvian sands were heard to hum in 1931.

All those who doubt that our early ancestors were capable of sophisticated intellectual, artistic and engineering achievements should read Corliss's *Ancient Man*. They will discover in it, for instance, an item on the Mayan highway that ran from Yaxuna to Coba. Built of stone and surfaced with cement, this nearly straight Mayan road, 62.5 miles long and 30 to 34 feet wide, is generally regarded as a magnificent engineering accomplishment.

Ancient Man also brings to light many high-tech artifacts thousands of years old that suggest knowledge of electrochemistry, metallurgy and analog computing. A reconstruction of a two-thousand-year-old wet-cell battery, for example, seems to indicate that such a device could have been used by silversmiths of Cleopatra's day for gold-plating jewelry.

This handbook of puzzling artifacts also presents dozens of cases of undeciphered writings. Ponder the puzzle of the painted pebbles: these neolithic or mesolithic relics, found in Europe, are painted with dots or strokes; some show conventional designs of trees, serpents and plants; others display about fourteen arbitrary characters resembling letters. These painted pebbles are remarkably similar to painted lima beans found on the sandy north coast of Peru. Behind such observations lie suspicions that not only was ancient man smarter than he has been given credit for, but that, judging from the great diffusion of inventions and cultural traits, he also traveled farther and earlier than conventional anthropologists have been willing to admit.

Corliss treats the more baffling aspects of human behavior in *The Unfathomed Mind.* It probes such topics as automatic writing, multiple personalities, apparitions and the prodigious capacity of the human brain. Did you know that a Persian king, Mithridates the Great, is said to have memorized the name of each soldier in his enormous army or that Racine could recite all the tragedies of Euripides? Another section probes the complex subject of mind-body interaction, an umbrella term that covers such phenomena as hysterical pregnancy, the placebo effect, and breast enlargement through hypnotic suggestion.

Of all the Sourcebooks, *Incredible Life* had perhaps the most potential for controversy. It deals, as might be expected, with the subject of unrecognized species. But more important is the thread of evidence running throughout the volume that poses challenges to Darwin's theory of evolution. "Evolution is a target," admits Corliss, "though not from a creationist standpoint. It simply questions whether the theory is doing the job properly."

Among the wealth of biological mysteries in *Incredible Life* are such items as the well-recognized biological phenomenon of synchronous flowering of bamboo plants. Some species of bamboo wait twenty to thirty years before flowering. Then, suddenly, they all flower, fruit and die at the same time. Even more remarkable is the fact that bamboos flower simultaneously even when transported half a world away from their native habitat. Clearly some kind of internal clock or calendar must trigger the flowering. But why would dwarf and fire-injured bamboos flower at the same time as healthy giants forty feet tall?

In the 1920s, eleven species of birds began prying open the wax tops of milk bottles set on the doorsteps of homes throughout Great Britain. How did they detect the presence of nourishment inside the bottles? Did each bird develop the habit on its own, or did they learn it from one another?

At the turn of the century several accounts appeared of humans shedding skin. In 1891, one member of the Chicago Medical Society observed a man who shed his skin every summer. He would be taken with feverish tremors for a period of twelve hours, during which his skin would turn red all over. It would then begin to peel, sometimes in great patches. "From the arms and legs it could be pulled off exactly like gloves or stockings," according to *Science*.

There is no denying the gee-whiz nature of many anomalies. Doubters like Corliss revel in them; creative minds find in anomalies the seeds of scientific revolutions. But Corliss is not antiscience; all the challenges raised in the Sourcebooks arise from the material itself, not from any belief he himself holds. "Instead of simply accepting nice, slick theories like evolution, relativity and continental drift," he says, "I think we should occasionally reexamine them to be sure they are not accepted just because they are so slick. And based upon the material I've collected, what I'm saying is I'm not so sure."

In fact, if Corliss were to have his way, there would be no theories at all in science. "There is much to be said for that idea," he says. "Theories imprint a whole view of the universe and make you look at everything through blinders. It is conceivable that you could do without theories altogether and use some sort of statistical method of evaluating past data and project the future from that."

Anomalies need the support of established scientists to acquire respectability. One of Corliss's entries, a piece on brontides, from the Greek meaning "thunder-like sounds," recently gained such support. Brontides are episodes of explosive noises of natural origin, first brought to the attention of the scientific community by George Darwin, son of Charles. Darwin *fils* wrote to *Nature* in 1895 describing the Barisal guns, unexplained explosive thuds that could be heard in the Ganges River delta. A quest for that original article unearthed a mass of references to similar rumblings in other parts of the world: the *mistpoeffers* (fog belchers) of Belgium, the Moodus sounds of Scotland and the Gouffre noises in Haiti.

At least one respected scientist apparently took note of Corliss's research and cited him in the list of references that appeared at the end of a report published in the prestigious journal *Science*. That man was Thomas Gold, the director of the Center for Radiophysics and Space Research at Cornell University, and the citation gave both Corliss and brontides the scientific stamp of approval.

The only criticism that can be justly leveled on the Sourcebooks is that they have a tendency to be indiscriminate collections of data. They touch on too many subjects to cover any one adequately. Many entries whet the appetite, but leave one ultimately unsatisfied. Yet one has to admire Corliss's courage in single-handedly attempting a project of such enormous scope. When he began, he had no idea that he would find so much material. Indeed, the Sourcebooks include but a fraction—about 15 percent—of what he uncovered. But the newest phase of the Sourcebook Project should help allay such criticism.

The Sourcebook Catalogs are a series of approximately two dozen "field guides" for the two thousand or so anomalies accumulated thus far. Each catalog includes a description of the phenomenon, its background, an evaluation of the data, an estimate of the anomaly's value to science, a list of similar and related phenomena and possible explanations, followed by examples, references, and illustrations. The first four volumes deal with geophysical anomalies.

"These catalogs are perhaps unique in the annals of science," says Corliss, "as I'm cataloging what is *not* known. It seems to me that any organized activity like science would have done this a long time ago. Instead we have encyclopedias and other books detailing what is known. Why the oversight?"

SCIENCE OF CYCLES

The cheapest single source of protein and fat on Earth is the soybean. It looks anything but impressive, and it doesn't taste like much before processing. But there is something curious about the fluctuations in the price of soybeans; plotted on a chart, two cycles appear. One peaks every 24.56 months and the other peaks every 38.6 months. Of course, the seasons have pronounced effect on soybean prices: you expect the price to go down when the crop comes in. It does, but trying to explain soybean prices by known causes like this only works about 70 percent of the time. It does not explain why soybean prices fluctuate cyclically the way they do.

Soybean prices are not alone in displaying this kind of cyclic behavior. Cycles, and the rhythms within them, seem to permeate all life and activity. Their presence is felt in everything from the beating of our hearts to the shifts in wind currents, and from the rise and fall of civilizations to the pulsations of distant stars.

Everything dances to the music of time. The population of Canadian lynx peaks every 9.6 years on the average; so do the populations of Atlantic salmon and chinch bugs in Illinois, the acreage of wheat harvested in the United States, and the incidence of heart disease in New England. But not all of nature marches to the same drummer. Plagues of mice, UFO sightings and cheese consumption reach peaks four years apart, while rainfall in England and shipbuilding in the United States come to a climax every fifty-four years.

Nature is prolific in her production of cyclic phenomena. "About one hundred new biological cycles are described every day," says biologist John Burns, the executive director of the Foundation for the Study of Cycles. "This makes it humanly impossible to keep track of them all." Yet the Foundation, which is located in a modest four-room suite in Pittsburgh, tries to do just that, and not only in biology. Since it was established in 1941, the Foundation has collected more than five hundred different examples of cycles from thirty-six different areas of knowledge, including economics, sociology, climatology, and astronomy.

Yet each branch of science has a tendency to view its cycles as unique and independent of similar patterns appearing in other areas of knowledge. For the most part biologists studying the breeding behavior of elephant seals have little interest in the fluctuation of cotton prices, and astronomers studying the pattern of sunspot recurrence could generally care less about the variations in admissions to mental hospitals. As a result, the study of the physical nature and character of cycles themselves tend to hover in a kind of scientific limbo.

One of the first people to look at cycles as unified symphony, rather than as isolated pictures-at-an-exhibition, was the late Edward R. Dewey. To Dewey, a Harvard economist who spent much of his life trying to make sense out of cyclical phenomena, the wide range of data suggested that only a truly interdisciplinary effort could ever lead to an understanding of these curious fluctuations. Having noticed that many cycles had characteristics in common, he began to wonder whether some unsuspected relationships might not exist between such completely different phenomena. But of one thing he seemed certain: Once you knew how a cycle had varied rhythmically in the past, you should be able to make an educated guess about the future. So he believed that cycles could help the farmer plant his crop, the doctor ward off epidemics, the weatherman make forecasts, and the stock market speculator make profits.

To investigate these notions Dewey established The Foundation for the Study of Cycles. The organization, which is devoted to the interdisciplinary study of rhythmic fluctuations in nature and society, acts as a clearinghouse for cycle research worldwide. Its small staff organizes international scientific conferences, sets up seminars for investors, and sponsors the *Journal of Interdisciplinary Cycle Research*. The Foundation also tries to formulate laws which govern the operation of cycles, and attempts to discover the causes of rhythmic fluctuations where the causes are not yet known. Since its inception, the Foundation has managed to attract people from all areas of science, and presently counts some 2,500 members from around the world.

The Foundation is primarily concerned with cycles that are both repetitive and rhythmic. A cycle is a chain of events that occurs in a set order and implies a return to the beginning from which it may begin again. When a cycle repeats, and there is a reasonably uniform period of time between repetitions, a cycle can then more accurately be called a rhythm. When the rhythm is repeated twelve to fifteen times, odds are that it is not due to chance. Such a rhythm may then be dynamic, meaning due to forces within the system itself, or forced, meaning that the regularity is imposed on the system from the outside. The heart beat is a dynamic rhythm. The tides are a forced rhythm.

At the heart of the Foundation's operations is a master file of thousands of three-by-five index cards, each listing a single cycle, and categorized by cycle length. On one card you will find data on human births—it has been claimed that they peak every five days. On another card, European wheat prices—they are said to reach a high every 5.96 years. International conflicts supposedly reach a maximum every fifty-seven years and the strength of world tides every 1,800 years. There is even a card for the expansion and contraction of the universe—once every fifty billion years. This cycle is obviously less well documented than some of the others, as it could hardly have passed the dozen-times-around test the Foundation requires to certify a repeating behavior as a rhythmic cycle.

To confirm an alleged cycle, the Foundation tries to obtain the data set on which it is based. Data sets are the lifeblood of the Foundation. "We have an enormous number of data sets," says Gertrude Shirk, a cycle sleuth with a special interest in statistics and economics. "They have been accumulated by historians and scholars from various disciplines, and the volume of information is growing all the time. Among others, we have numbers for the flood stages of the Nile River beginning in A.D. 622. We have a record of iron production in Sweden going back to the Middle Ages. And we have a data set on the geomagnetic index going back to 1868."

The Foundation tries to extract cycles from these data sets with the help of a statistical technique called time series analysis. A time series is a numerical record of fluctuating behavior over time, and time series analysis attempts to separate out the cycle from other components in a time series that sometimes tend to obscure it. These include trend, or the prevailing tendency up or down, and noise, or interference, which is random.

"You have to know what you are doing in time series analysis so that you do not inadvertently color or distort your results," says Shirk, who has put in thirty-one years at the Foundation. She spends much of her time immersed in data sets. "It's hard to look at a chart and not see cycles," she admits. "It's a sort of occupational hazard. But you can never make any assumptions about what might be there. Science normally works from a theory, but in cycle research there is no theory. That's not to say that it's not scientific, just that it makes it harder for people to understand."

After identifying a cycle, the Foundation is, of course, eager to understand what causes it—and here often finds itself facing a mystery. "For instance," says Shirk, "you can explain about 90 percent of the motion of copper prices by such things as the size of the copper stockpile, the delivery of the metal, and so on. But all this will not explain why copper prices have a cycle around nine years in length. Even after you explain the changes in cycle by cause, you often cannot explain its rhythm. That means that our knowledge of events and behaviors is partial and that there may be things going on that we don't know about."

The Foundation brings together information from many diverse disciplines in the hope of recognizing common patterns among cycles. In comparative studies, many cycles exhibit similar periods and appear to vary simultaneously. Dewey uncovered sixteen phenomena with four-year periods, ten with 5.9-year periods, thirty-eight with six-year periods, thirty-seven with eight-year periods, thirty-one with nine-year periods, among others. Though Dewey was well aware that similarities in cycle periods could occur by sheer coincidence, he thought the fact that so many cycles seemed to act in synchrony, regardless of phenomena or discipline involved, was powerful evidence that he was dealing with meaningful rather than random behavior. "The suggestion is thus inescapable," he wrote, "that there may be hitherto unsuspected environmental forces which affect terrestrial affairs and determine the time of the ups and downs of many phenomena of interest and concern to mankind."

But observers have always been very critical of attempts to correlate unrelated phenomena, such as weather variables and psychological moods, for example. "Our statistical methods are still too crude to decipher what such correlations might mean," says Dr. Arne Sollberger, a professor of physiology at Southern Illinois University Medical School and a co-editor of the *Journal of Interdisciplinary Cycle Research*. "The reason is simply that the relationship between the two variables is much too noisy. Unfortunately, all cycles go up and down, so there is almost always a statistically significant correlation between any of them, though it is often a nonsense correlation. We must guard against the dangers of seeing cycles where there are none. Biorhythms, for instance, are sheer numerology. The rhythms that believers in biorhythms postulate have never been found."

Whether or not cyclic phenomena have a common cause, it is undeniable that a knowledge of cycles can be useful for predicting and manipulating the future. In recent years, chronobiologists have begun to explore the medical applications of biological rhythms, which are distinct from biorhythms, and their knowledge is now being put to work in fields such as endocrinology, immunology, anesthesiology and oncology.

In the kind of simple skin test used to check a patient's response to a foreign substance, for example, immunologists have begun to take into account circadian, or approximately daily, rhythms. It is now known that when histamine is injected beneath the skin, it produces a red patch that varies in size depending on the time of day the shot is given. Anesthesiologists, too, are taking cycles into consideration. They found that in most patients, the drug lidocaine will cause maximum numbness of the front teeth if it is injected between one o'clock and three o'clock in the afternoon.

Allergists also have discovered that the body's natural rhythms, during which time hormone levels rise and fall, can increase or decrease a drug's potency. It seems that some anti-allergy drugs are more effective when taken immediately after waking rather than in the late afternoon or evening. In fact, the time at which most any drug is taken can greatly modify the result. Insulin, for instance, has been shown to be lethal when given to hamsters at night, but harmless when the same dose is administered during the day.

The application of cycles in the treatment of cancer has also shown great promise. Dr. Lawrence Scheving, a chronobiologist at the University of Arkansas College of Medicine, has conducted some groundbreaking lab studies on the application of circadian cycles to the treatment of cancer. Scheving's studies indicate that some chemotherapies may be more effective if administered when the cancer cells are dividing. Because some tumors have circadian rhythms of cell division differing from those of the healthy surrounding tissue, Scheving suggests that therapy be applied at the time of day when it will be most toxic to the tumor cells and least harmful to noncancerous tissue. The idea of timed treatment is not a cure for cancer, Scheving warns, but such a chronobiological advantage may one day lead to a better understanding of the mechanism and causes of cancer.

Climatology is another, very different, science that is taking note of cycles. Dr. Charles Stockton, a hydrologist at the Laboratory of Tree Ring Research at the University of Arizona, has made extensive studies of tree rings in an effort to understand the history of climatic variations west of the Mississippi. Like many other scientists, Stockton had not gone looking for cycles but found one anyway. His tree ring samples indicate a strong twenty-two year drought cycle, and he believes that careful planning is necessary to avoid the next severe water shortage, due around the year 2000.

His data also suggest an interesting correlation. Except for some decades in the mid-to-late 1800s, the worse droughts seem to have come two years after the sunspot minimum in the Hale cycle. This twenty-two-year cycle, composed of two eleven-year sunspot cycles, occurs when the sun's magnetic polarity reverses from north to south or vice versa. Along with other scientists, Stockton is now pursuing the question of how the sun may have an effect on the weather.

Although this sort of applied cycle research is relatively recent, cycles themselves have been recognized since the earliest times. Ecclesiastes spoke of the wind that "turns again and again, resuming its rounds," and Shakespeare wrote of "a tide in the affairs of men, which taken at the flood, leads on to fortune." But a formal, scientific interest in cycles dates back only about a century. In 1891, Eduard Bruckner proposed the existence of a thirty-five-year cycle in European weather, and before the turn of the century Ernest Thompson Seton, the American naturalist, drew attention to the rhythmic variations in animal populations.

The seed from which the Foundation for the Study of cycles itself grew was planted in the fall of 1929. Just a few weeks before the world fell apart amid crashing stock prices, a bright young Harvard graduate in economics and sociology named Edward R. Dewey took a job with the Hoover administration. After a hitch at the Bureau of the Census as collector of statistics on industrial marketing, he went on to become the chief economic analyst at the Bureau of Foreign and Domestic Commerce. It was in this position, he recalls in his book *Cycles: The Mysterious Forces that Trigger Events,* that he was assigned the task of discovering "why a prosperous and growing nation had been reduced to a frightened mass of humanity selling apples on street corners and waiting in line for bowls of watery soup."

No one could figure out why the Great Depression had occured—Dewey included. Every economist he spoke to had a different explanation, and his faith in economics languished, until several years and several jobs later, when he met Chapin Hoskins, a former managing editor of *Forbes,* who introduced him to the theory of business cycles. In 1937, with Hoskins doing the forecasting, Dewey began selling businesses on the benefits of the cycle theory; his pitch was that it could help a company forecast sales, production costs, profits and so forth. Soon they had a client list that included such firms as Consolidated Edison and Lehman Brothers.

Bitten by the cycle bug, Dewey spent much of his free time in the library, trying to find out what was then known about repeating behavior. One day he chanced upon the proceedings of a conference on biological cycles that had been held in July

1931. It had taken place at the summer residence of a Boston financier and wildlife fancier named Copley Amory, and was attended by some of the world's leading biologists, zoologists, and physiologists. Their papers made a great impression on Dewey; they told of cycles among Canadian lynx, snowshoe rabbits, Atlantic salmon and other species. If cycles occurred in biology as well as in economics, Dewey concluded, then cycles might turn out to be a detective story of cosmic proportions.

Within weeks he had contacted Amory and proposed to establish a foundation that would further the study of cycles. Amory jumped at the idea and even kicked in $500 to get the Foundation on its feet. The charter executive committee included such distinguished scientists as Julian Huxley, then secretary of the Zoological Society of London, and Harlow Shapley, then director of the Harvard Observatory. The very first dues-paying member was the then Representative and later Senator Everett Dirksen of Illinois.

During its first decade, from 1941 to 1951, the Foundation did little more than continue the work in economics that Dewey had begun with Hoskins. Problems arose, however, as corporations, keen on competition, wanted the Foundation to keep its findings secret. To escape this corporate muzzle, Dewey transformed the Foundation into what it is today: a nonprofit, tax-exempt, membership-only scientific body, affiliated with the University of Pittsburgh.

Today, as in Dewey's time, it devotes much of its time to trying to make sense of business and economic cycles, in part because so much data is available on economic matters, but also, no doubt, because many of its dues-paying members are interested with making money. So the Foundation keeps close tabs on all business cycles. Among the business cycles that have been alleged over the years are the forty-one-month cycle in stock prices, the 17.75-year cycle in cotton prices, and the 18.3-year building construction cycle. The most reliable economic cycles seem to be those based on specific segments of industry rather than on the broad sweep of events. Yet the most notorious economic cycle of all time is the broad 48-60-year cycle known as the Kondratieff long-wave.

Looking back to the eighteenth century, the late Russian economist Nikolai Dimitriyevich Kondratieff noticed that human affairs had always been subjected to great waves of prosperity and adversity. He began wondering about the great tides in economic affairs and calculated that these peaks and troughs fluctuated in cycles which were fifty-four years long on the average. If Kondratieff's pattern holds true, the last upswing would have peaked in the 1970s around the time of the OPEC oil crunch, meaning that we are now in the full throes of a major downswing. Though he could never explain why these great waves rose and fell, the belief in economic cycles has persisted.

The views expressed by Federal Reserve Board chairman Paul Volcker in *The Rediscovery of the Business Cycle* illustrate the attraction that a cyclic view of business still has for some prominent economists. "The evidence . . . seems to me pretty clear that there is some tendency toward swings in the tempo and mood of business activity over relatively long periods of time," wrote Volcker, "say periods of ten to twenty years." To Volcker, the 1973–1975 recession demonstrated the existence of these business cycles. He also noted a shorter cycle of three to four years, which he thought might be related to inventory fluctuations. Volcker, however, saw no convincing evidence of a degree of regularity in the long cycles. He concluded that government monetary actions could be used to avoid extreme swings in economic cycles.

It is precisely this sort of action, based on a knowledge of cycles, that Dewey always promoted. Yet, curiously, until his death in 1978 at the age of eighty-two, Dewey concentrated much of the Foundation's resources on a quixotic search for a single cause for all cycles. For a time, he toyed with such notions as sunspots, and planetary alignments to explain cycles, but ultimately he rejected them. "He died frustrated," says executive director Burns. "He realized that he had not been able to find a cause, nor had he been able to propose a substantial, general theory of cycles. He had accumulated various clues and shreds of evidence, but the overall picture had not been brought together in a sense that was at all satisfactory to him. But he did leave a trail that others could follow."

The Foundation nearly lapsed into obscurity following Dewey's death, perhaps from the weight of the enormous task he left behind, perhaps from the realization that even a complete understanding of cycles would never yield the much-sought-after magic formula of life. In any case, the Foundation is well aware that cycles are far from being an exact science. Shirk points out that even in the best of cycles there is wobble, and Dewey was well aware of that. "We assume that the cyclic forces are regular," he wrote many years ago, "partly because they 'ought' to be regular and partly because we don't know how to deal with them unless they are regular."

Dewey realized that the study of cycles was a young science. He compared its progress to the early days of astronomy, when it was thought that the Sun and all the planets moved around the Earth in huge circles. Then Copernicus came along and put the Sun at the center of things, and Kepler explained the circles were actualy ellipses. "If we only knew enough," Dewey argued, "some of the irregularities of the cycles might be predicted too. What we need is a Copernicus and a Kepler in cycle study."

Yet it was Dewey's firm belief that the field of cycles, despite its shortcomings, was an area worthy of scientific study. He was convinced that cycles held implications for science that were both startling and fundamental. If such order, regularity, and pattern exists in phenomena previously thought to be unrelated, he reasoned, then there must be a much greater interrelationship within nature than has ever been realized. But such knowledge, he knew, could yield bitter fruit. In a cyclic view of the world, we become pawns in the great waves, cycles, and forces of history and nature. He wondered if we might not be a mere collection of corks bobbing up and down on a vast ocean beset by great waves of bewildering complexity. He concluded that we were not, but only if we could recognize our condition—the influence of cycles on our lives.

CHARTING TOMORROWS

Every age has its soothsayers, and ours is no different in that respect. But modern times would never have bestowed its good graces on the ancient art of prophecy without the obligatory facelift. The tea leaves and crystal balls just had to go, and with them went the oracles and seers of yesteryear.

In its modern incarnation, the art of prophesy has become the science of forecasting. Today, the practice of guessing what lies around the next bend in time is being performed by engineers, computer scientists, economists, historians, and businessmen. At their service are hundreds of sophisticated new forecasting techniques based upon history, mathematics, and expert opinion.

Only the forecasters' clients have remained the same over the centuries. As always, it is the power elite that seeks information about the future, and today that includes not only the government and the military, but many of the Fortune 500 companies as well. What this all means, of course, is a tremendous change at the bottom line. The old nickel-and-dime business of looking into the future has blossomed into a thriving, multi-billion dollar industry.

At no time in history has our desire to anticipate the future burned so strongly in our minds. "Our concern for the future has increased because the future has become so much less predictable," explains Roy Amara, president of the Institute for the Future (IFTF), in Menlo Park, California. "You see, people are not going to be interested in the future if the conditions tomorrow are going to be essentially the same as they have been today. They only become interested when the uncertainties about the conditions tomorrow increases."

The rapid social, political and technological changes that characterize the present—and the uncertainties these create for the future—have sent businessmen and politicians scurrying to the altars of our modern-day visionaries. Decision makers and planners want to make sure that the actions they take today will be in line with what is likely to happen tomorrow. "The future influences the present just as much as the past," said the nineteenth-century German philosopher Friedrich Nietzche. Never have his words rung so true.

This voracious new appetite for information about the future means that the science of forecasting is being applied to just about every subject under the sun, even those beyond it. Forecasters are now predicting employee turnover, water demand, fertility rates, traffic flow, sports performance, milk production, and life expectancy, as well as the spread of epidemics, the winners of political elections, the demand for new products, the outcome of football games, the trajectory of comets, and naturally, the weather.

Yet it would be foolish to oversell the ability of this new science to forecast complex events accurately and completely. The process of transforming prediction from an art to a science has just begun. "A scientific attitude has developed in forecasting only within the past twenty-five years," notes J. Scott Armstrong, one of the founders of the International Institute of Forecasters and a professor of marketing at the University of Pennsylvania's Wharton School in Philadelphia.

At the moment forecasting might best be described as a soft science, like psychology and economics. "It's a science in the sense that forecasting now uses systematic procedures, which produces repeatable results," says Andrew Lipinski, a senior research fellow at IFTF. He defines forecasting as "a way of presenting the best possible information there is about the future." Since its founding in 1968, the IFTF has pioneered in the development of forecasting tools which it has used to help industry and government plan their long-term futures.

Not all ventures into forecasting are equally successful. "Forecasting is most difficult in the area of politics," says IFTF president Amara. "A little less difficult perhaps, is social forecasting. Next along the scale comes economics, followed by weather forecasting. Then there's technological forecasting. And at the top of the scale, what we are best at, is physical forecasting." This type of forecasting applies to areas in the physical sciences in which we have a complete understanding of the causes involved, allowing us to make very accurate predictions. Because we understand the movement of the Sun, for example, we know when it will rise and set every day for as long as the Sun and the Earth exist as they do today.

The ability of modern forecasters to see into the future falls far short of the epoch-spanning forecasts of ancient seers like Nostradamus. Present-day forecasting concerns itself primarily with short-term estimates, meaning up to a couple of years away. This is the most dependable range of time in which to make a forecast, as the changes which must be anticipated are not as numerous, and their interactions not as complex as they would be over longer time spans.

Yet long-term forecasting still attracts the greatest attention, the most important decision makers, and naturally, the most money. When forecasters talk about long-term predictions, however, they mean no more than about fifteen years ahead. "Our level of understanding decreases very rapidly after that," says Amara, "and the uncertainty factor becomes so great that the forecasts are not terribly credible for someone who wants to use them to make decisions in the present."

The "lead time" of a forecast is often imposed by the nature of the subject being studied. "In some instances," Amara continues, "it becomes absolutely necessary to make statements about the state of affairs twenty-five or more years into the future. A case in point is whether fossil fuel burning will raise the level of carbon dioxide in the atmosphere enough to cause appreciable warming, and whether such a climate change would alter the global ecology. If this should become a life threatening situation, we would like to know about it well in advance, because it's going to take us from twenty-five to forty years to rearrange our energy production patterns."

Just how far ahead forecasters can see into the future actually is not a matter of time at all. "Forecasting approaches don't really look ahead in time," explains Selwyn Enzer, the associate director of the Center for Futures Research, located at the University of Southern California in Los Angeles. "The real issue is change. When you try to anticipate the future and the environment is generally stable and unchanging, it's very easy to predict hundreds of years ahead. But in a turbulent environment, it's very hard to predict a long time ahead. So it's wrong to say, for example, that forecasters have a twenty-year vision. What we can say is that we can see through one, two, or three cycles of change. In chess, you might say that you can see six moves ahead. How much time that is depends on how fast you play. Cycles of change are the limiting factor; after two or three cycles the puzzle becomes too complex to anticipate."

During the past fifty years forecasters have developed a number of powerful new tools to probe the future. Some two hundred techniques of forecasting are known to exist, though many of them are no more than slight variations on a handful of methods that are in general use. The five major approaches to forecasting are known as barometric, extrapolative, causal, simulative, and judgmental.

Barometric forecasts examine the present to reveal the future. To produce the forecasts in his best-selling book, *Megatrends*, John Naisbitt used a barometric method known as content analysis. This method picks the trend, or the direction in which a system is moving, by simply analyzing the fluctuations in the amount of space newspapers give to each of a number of topics of concern.

Still the most common way to generate a forecast, however, is by extrapolation. It is known as the technique of applied history because the method assumes that the patterns of the past will continue into the future. Most extrapolation uses a kind of eyeball approach. A simple straight line, for instance, will give you a reasonable estimate of a city's population five years down the road, if you know, for example, that the city's population has grown 2 percent a year for each of the past ten years. More complex patterns may project themselves as curves.

When the causes of a system are known, extremely precise predictions can be made. Econometric forecasting is the most widely known causal method of forecasting, though as we all know, the method is far from creating an entirely accurate model of the behavior of a national economy. Econometrics relies on good economic data, which exists, assumes that the process is stable, which it isn't, and then proceeds to extract very scientifically the relationships among the various factors known to affect a nation's economy. The set of mathematical equations that result constitute a model which allows economists to make certain predictions about the future state of that economy.

All methods of forecasting involve the transformation of existing data into simulations, or models of the future. The wind tunnel model of a new airplane, which is used to predict how the full-scale version of that airplane will operate in real-life, is an example of how mechanical models are used to predict the future. A computer simulation of the Earth's atmosphere, which NASA is using to assess the impact of human activity on the future composition and chemistry of the atmosphere, is a mathematical type of model.

When the underlying mechanism is not fully understood, metaphorical models, or analogies, are useful in forecasting. Freeman Dyson, a physicist at Princeton's Institute of Advanced Studies and one of the nimblest thinkers of our time, used an historical analogy to predict that space colonization would not take place until the year 2085. Dyson arrived at that forecast after calculating that 128 years elapsed between Columbus's discovery of America and the Mayflower's establishment of the first permanent colony in the New World. He then assumed that all government-sponsored projects probably take about the same amount of time to become accessible to the public and simply added 128 years to the year 1957, the date of the first Sputnik shot.

Yet another simulation model is the game. One type of game used as a predictive technique is role-playing, in which the interactions between game "players" is taken to represent a real-world social event. Professor J. Scott Armstrong of the Wharton Business School used the role-playing technique to predict the outcome of a variety of conflict situations, and found that the predictions of the outcome of the conflict situations by the role-players was far more accurate than the predictions of those who did not participate in the game.

No method of forecasting, regardless of its technical sophistication, can be entirely free of the exercise of human judgment. One category of forecasting methods, in fact, is based entirely on educated intuition. These are the judgmental methods, and they are the most widely used techniques in forecasting.

One of the world's most respected futurists, the late Herman Kahn, was probably the foremost practitioner of the judgmental method known as "genius forecasting." His ability to estimate, assess and predict various aspects of the future was based largely on intuition and depended a good deal on luck and insight. To improve on individual judgments, forecasters have developed consensus methods of forecasting. These are based on the notion that the judgment of a number of informed people is likely to be better than the judgment of a single individual.

Scenarios represent another kind of judgmental forecasting. The method begins by asking "What if such-and-such occurs?" and then proceeds to describe a view of the future based on that initial speculation. This method's greatest strength, its ability to convince, is based largely on the storyteller's ability. This is also its greatest weakness. "If you are good at storytelling," says Armstrong, "you can build a scenario with a lot of very unlikely events, link them together in a graphic and plausible way, and make something very implausible appear likely to people."

The million-dollar question, of course, is how good are these forecasting methods? It turns out that when forecasters attempt to give precise, single-number forecasts about the future, no matter what method they use, the batting averages are not particularly impressive. "It's a losing game," says forecaster Andrew Lipinski. "People hang themselves on single numbers."

To avoid the embarrassment of constantly being wrong, forecasters have turned increasingly to probability forecasting, which takes into account the distribution of uncertainty involved in making a prediction. Probabilities can be assigned to all forecasts, regardless of the forecasting technique employed. Much of the research done on forecasting methodologies in the past few years has been devoted to quantifying the subjective or judgmental methods of forecasting. One way to do this is by asking respondents how certain they are of their opinions, so that the respondents themselves can be judged on the basis of their relative expertise. Ideally, this process transforms everyone into perfect assessors and their opinions into perfect assessments.

"I think forecasters have become humbler about the efficacy of their methods," says Amara, "in part because the world has become more complex and more uncertain, and in part because clients of forecasters have held their feet to the fire. I think that the only responsible forecasters today are those who try to capture the degree of uncertainty that is present, rather than try to suppress it by making point forecasts about any variable. Forecasts must be accompanied by probability figures. That lesson was learned many decades ago, but forecasters are only human and they like to be seduced by those who pay homage to them."

Single number forecasts assume that the future, in a sense, already exists, that it is predetermined. "But suppose," says futures researcher Selwyn Enzer, "that tomorrow is an uncertain thing, and that it depends on two different kinds of uncertainties: those which are beyond our present understanding, like earthquakes, and uncertainties of human action. If those are true uncertainties then tomorrow is not predestined to be anything, but depends on how the process resolves itself. Only by understanding the process can we learn anything about the possibilities. That's where futures research is at today."

The focus of forecasting appears to have undergone a dramatic change in the past decade. *Predictions* of the future have largely been replaced by *studies* of the future. This change is the result of a new view which holds, according to Enzer, "that the future contains key uncertainties that cannot be eliminated by prophecy, but that the alternative ways these uncertainties might be resolved can be analyzed and described."

The various paths these uncertainties might take as they are resolved are known as "alternative futures." These can be viewed as the various faces that appear on a pair of dice. "The futures researcher," continues Enzer, "is concerned with anticipating the various faces that may appear on the dice and estimating the probability of each outcome. Forecasters are usually concerned with predicting the outcome or the most likely outcome, but rarely all of the outcomes and their probabilities."

The biggest roadblock facing futures researchers today, insists Enzer, is that users of future information shun uncertainty. They still want that one answer that says this is what the future will be. Enzer believes that users will have to change the way they function in order to use information about the future properly.

"Once they come to realize that the future cannot be known in advance with any degree of certainty," he explains, "that the future is actually a dynamic environment where different things can happen, they will begin to think of all the uncertainties, never ruling out a possibility, and prepare for all of them. They must, in short, act like a field general. They may still assume that one future is most likey to occur, but they should have their sentries posted for the others and be ready for them if they occur."

Enzer calls this the management of change. It seems to be here that forecasting will prove most useful in the future, rather than in the essentially futile attempts to give precise predictions about what lies around the next bend in time.